CANCER PROOF

7 NATURAL WAYS TO LIVE CANCER-FREE

DR. HEATHER PAULSON

Cancer Proof

7 Natural Ways to Live Cancer Free

Dr. Heather Paulson, ND, FABNO

This book is intended to supplement, not replace, the advice of a trained health professional. If you know or think you have a health problem, you should consult with a health professional. The author and publisher specifically disclaim any liability, loss, or risk, personal or otherwise, that is incurred as a consequence, directly or indirectly, of the use and application of any contents of this book.

DISCLAIMER

✳—✳—✳

A lthough the author and publisher have made every effort to ensure that the information in this book was correct at press time, the author and publisher do not assume and hereby disclaim any liability to any party for any loss, damage, or disruption caused by errors or omissions, whether such errors or omissions result from negligence, accident, or any other cause.

This book is not intended to substitute for the medical advice of physicians. The reader should regularly consult a physician in matters relating to his/her health and particularly with respect to any symptoms that may require diagnosis or medical attention.

This book is written as a source of information only. The information in this book should by no means be considered a substitute for the advice of a qualified medical professional, who should always be consulted before beginning any health program.

DEDICATION

※ — ※ — ※

This book is dedicated to one of my greatest teachers, my Dad, Glenn Paulson. Your memory fuels everything I do.

CONTENTS

※—※—※

INTRODUCTION:
CHANGE IS POSSIBLE

❋—❋—❋

If there were a medication that could be prescribed to reduce your risk of cancer by 50%, would you take it? What if I told you that you already have access to it and that it doesn't come from a doctor? With simple and easy lifestyle changes you could potentially reduce your risk of cancer by 50%.

Now, I know you've been through a lot. You have probably read or heard more than enough medical terms that only a professional could comprehend. I know how tough it is to not understand how to take charge of your own health. I remember what it was like to feel totally lost and confused when it comes to cancer.

But making sense of cancer doesn't have to be difficult. You can easily understand what it takes to live a healthy and fulfilled life. Better yet, living a cancer-prevention lifestyle doesn't have to include crazy juice fasts, drastic moves, or heroic measures. And if that's the case, wouldn't that be awesome?!

I know that our family would have loved to have this information when my dad was going through his colon cancer journey. When we were in doctor appointments, reading websites, and sifting through research, it seemed like everyone was speaking a different language. In fact, when I went to medical school, I looked at my time spend there as a 4-year long course in a foreign language. Which seems crazy, right? Because how can our own bodies be such a foreign place to us? No specialist knows your body better than you do. And yet, we can't even find the right words to talk about our bodies and our health.

When you arrive at the hospital or doctor's office, you are not alone in feeling like you're entering some strange country where you don't know the language, the rituals, and the culture. You are not alone in being lost in the different diets, supplements, and 'cures' for cancer. We have all been there.

We have all felt that overwhelming sense of... *What did that doctor say? Wait...the nutritionist wants me to do what? Isn't there a cancer road map to help me find my way through this?*

Well, here it is!

Cancer Proof is that road map.

When we clear away the fancy medical terms and look at bigger studies that focus on even bigger questions, cancer is simple. Not only is it simple, there are only a handful things that have been shown to reduce cancer risk, recurrence, and growth.

That's why I wrote this book to help you understand your body, learn the simple changes that can make a huge impact, and ultimately get you living a vibrant, healthy life connected to love and a sense of fulfillment — a life that, right now, you might not think is possible. This is the road map I wish my family had before my dad died of colon cancer. It's the road map I started creating over a decade ago when my husband was diagnosed with lymphoma. And now, it can be your road map too!

When I devised the very beginnings of *Cancer Proof*, we used the principles during and after my husband's lymphoma and he was able to run a half marathon just six months after chemo finished. Pretty amazing, right? (More of that story in the exercise chapter).This hasn't just happened for my husband. I have seen countless men and women accomplish things they never thought they would be able to do after working through these *Cancer Proof* methods with me. Things like:

- Getting rid of cancer treatment side effects

- Losing weight

- Having increased energy

- Starting to exercise… and keeping with it

- Clearing brain fog

- Feeling like themselves again.

You're probably thinking: *That's great for those people, but I can't have those results. It's probably going to be too hard, and I just don't have the time or energy.* Maybe you're still in a cloud of cancer information or overwhelmed by where your life is right now, and it's hard to commit to beginning a change. It's probably feeling difficult for you at the moment because of all the time spent at doctor's appointments. Those doctors might have even said that changes don't matter. Perhaps it's your family that isn't ready for change, or someone has told you that you can't change, because you have so much happening and so many other commitments.

It's challenging when you haven't found the right person to guide you through a time of change, even though you have been looking. You may have felt like you couldn't trust the information out there on the internet about natural medicine and cancer. It's even possible that you're reading this when you haven't been diagnosed with cancer and don't feel any urgency to make changes in your life.

The truth is that anything could be reason enough to stop you from making changes if you let it be. But look what can happen if you allow change into your life...

"I feel so good, and am very grateful. I have a new life... finally. THANK YOU ♥" ~ Cindy, Arizona

"I have learned balance in my food choices and how to stay centered throughout the day." ~ Margaretha, New

York

"I am living again 100% of the time instead of just treading water and existing." ~ Julie, Colorado

"I am challenging myself more to say 'yes' to life, explore healthier cooking, and to REST!" ~ Anna, California

Why I studied cancer

I know what's it's like to be overwhelmed by cancer. See, when my dad was diagnosed with colon cancer, I was only 18 years old and had just moved to Santa Barbara to start my university studies in aquatic biology. While I was in the biology research library studying ocean and river systems, I would frequently end up in the medical research section reading everything I could get my hands on about cancer. I didn't have a medical background. I didn't understand cancer research. I was studying fish, aquaculture, kelp forests, and sea cucumbers. That had nothing to do with words like *angiogenesis*, *p53*, *tyrosine kinase*, and the *human genome...*

If you have ever tried to understand exactly how to prevent or treat cancer, you know that it can be so complicated. Most of us get lost somewhere between eating sugar and cancer genetics. Like you, my family wanted to turn to diet, supplements, herbs, and a whole host of natural therapies for my dad. I became the lead cancer researcher for my family at only 18 years old. We got lost in all the complicated details. So lost, in fact, that we ended up not being able to implement or change anything while my dad was alive.

While I was sitting with my dad during the last days of his life, his doctors recommended his first diet change. After five years of asking for diet suggestions! Unfortunately the nutrition change they recommended was that he should be getting his meals through a tube because he could no longer eat solid food. I was outraged that this was the only way his doctors would weigh in on nutrition.

In that moment, at just 22 years old and on my path to a great career in marine biology, I decided to stop what I was doing and become a doctor. I could not allow another person or family to suffer and be confused the way my family had been during the past five years. I was determined to figure out cancer.

My dad never got to hear this declaration or see the impact his life has on so many people. He was no longer in a verbal state when I made this internal declaration, and the quiet moments felt too precious. I didn't want to interrupt our last moments together with decisions that he would no longer be part of. So I just sat there holding his hand while he transitioned from this life and slowly unwound from his physical body.

With a sense of purpose and determination, I prepared to attend medical school. Since I had been studying fish and marine mammals, I went back to university to take a couple of pre-med classes so I could start understanding humans a little better. My family was both skeptical and supportive. All my life, I had only talked about studying the ocean… And now this girl that passes out at the sight of blood is going to medical school? You could understand their caution!

Flash forward to over a decade later. With a dedication to my dad's legacy in my heart, I persevered through medical school, an oncology residency, passing the oncology board exam, and speaking at international conventions to doctors and healthcare providers trying to understand cancer. In all this time, I never forgot my declaration to make cancer understandable for everyone. I have never lost my connection to that 18-year-old girl so bewildered by cancer in the biology library. This declaration of a young woman grieving because of cancer has turned into *Cancer Proof*. I want you and your family to have what I never had the chance to give to my dad.

Getting the most out of this book

Let me be clear. There is nothing on this planet at this time, not me, no healer, no medication, no diet or natural supplement that can guarantee a cure to cancer. Personally, when people talk about 'cancer cures', I turn off and walk the other way. Cancer has so many layers to it. And cancer cells turn on and persist for so many different reasons. Cancer can be started from genes, environment, hormones, emotional states, soul contracts, and everything in between. So please, if someone talks to you about being able to cure your cancer, use discernment.

I wish I knew the secret to completely ridding our planet of cancer. It would save so much heartache and pain if I did. Including my own heartache, pain, and loss. Of course, I can't make that happen. However, I *have* been using these *Cancer Proof* steps in my practice with my patients with great results and I've heard stories that are beyond my expectations.

This book is not a compilation of natural cancer cures. This book is about empowering you with the tools you need to create a lifestyle that prevents cancer growth. And yes, it might even reduce cancer growth. *Cancer Proof* is compiled from almost two decades of research and lessons I've learned in my clinical practice, through seeing what people *really* need and helping thousands of people with cancer.

Over a decade of practicing naturopathic oncology, I've seen certain patterns and paths that my patients have taken that led them to no longer fearing cancer. Letting go of fear is one way to *Cancer Proof* your life, to not let cancer occupy your brain space, every moment, every thought. That means, even if you still have tumors in your body, you can *Cancer Proof* your life.

I believe that purely focusing on cancer cures is focusing on the wrong issue. Instead of staring at a disease process, 'fighting' it, and winning a battle, I like to help people focus on living a life they love (with or without disease), feeling healthy with plenty of energy, being unlimited by external circumstances, and being surrounded by fulfilling relationships. This may stand counter to what other health practitioners have been telling you. They want to help you fight, survive the fight, and try to pick up the pieces afterwards.

But what if cancer care could be a process of peace, non-violence, health, and self-care? I stand for this as the future of cancer care. That is why my husband Phil and I co-founded The Paulson Center. When Phil was diagnosed with cancer, our experience was full of stress, uncomfortable environments, and a lack of acknowledging the human who was going through the process of healing. We wanted to create a space that's peaceful, cozy, loving, and focused on wellness and health no matter what stage of cancer you have. From prevention to Stage 4.

We believe that the future of cancer care stands in acknowledging you and your individuality. Coming to peace with every cell in your body. Embracing detoxification practices. Incorporating spiritual and traditional healing practices. If this sounds like what you may be looking for in your life, you are ready to embrace the *Cancer Proof* lifestyle.

You have a choice right now: ignore cancer and do nothing; fight cancer like it's an enemy; or use cancer as a pivot point towards personal transformation. If you put into practice the steps of the *Cancer Proof* lifestyle, you will be able to experience greater wholeness and healing, embrace your life more fully no matter what your disease stage, and have a simple strategy for becoming *Cancer Proof*. I'd like to invite you to not just read this book, but look for practices you can put into motion immediately.

For your first step towards living a *Cancer Proof* life, come join our community of support. In this group you will be able to ask questions, share recipes, give exercise tips, and have support from others living a *Cancer Proof* life! I'll be keeping an eye on this group and making sure you are getting the support you need. Just go to https://www.facebook.com/groups/greatlifeplan/ and join this community of support.

Cancer is a personal journey, but the people we meet along the road make all the difference. Sometimes this means creating deeper connections to friends and family members already in our lives. Other times, this means support from people sitting next to you in the infusion room. I'm glad to meet you on your path. It is an honor to be here for support, information, and maybe even a little inspiration. I look forward to getting to know each other.

May you be blessed with healing and transformation.

To your health,

Dr. Heather Paulson

CHAPTER 1:
KNOW YOURSELF

✳ — ✳ — ✳

Let's start with what makes your cancer or cancer risk different from everyone else, because that's how you'll start to see that this *Cancer Proof* lifestyle is a personal journey.

In this chapter, you'll learn:

- what you can control (and what you can't)

- what lab tests are out there and what they'll tell you

- key genetic markers for cancer

- lab work that identifies your unique characteristics

- genetics and cancer risk.

You are unique

No two people are exactly alike; not even identical twins are exactly the same. In the same way, no two cancers are alike. You have different risk factors, physiology, and genes that uniquely set up your cancer risk. Not only do these issues influence cancer risk, but also how cancer grows once you have been diagnosed.

The first step in knowing your cancer risk and what makes your cancer unique is to find out about your personal and family medical history. Certain medical conditions like diabetes and high blood pressure, and lifestyle habits like smoking, drinking, and sleeping less than 7 or more than 9 hours per night all are known to increase the risk of having cancer. Vitamin deficiencies in dietary intake such as vitamin D, folate, selenium, vitamin E, and zinc can also increase your cancer risk. Some of these nutrients are only protective when you get them from food, and might actually be harmful when taken as a supplement. So it's helpful to know *exactly* which nutrients to focus on in our diets.

If you're unsure about your family history, reach out and connect to those who might know. Be sure to ask about cancer history, diabetes, cardiovascular disease, environmental exposures, and blood disorders. If this is not available to you, consider genomic/genetic testing such as www.23andme.com, which can give broad overviews about your health.

While at your doctor's appointment, make sure you follow through with recommended screenings such as colonoscopies, pap smears, mole checks, prostate and testicular exams, or mammograms. You cannot underestimate the healing power of prevention! Proper screening is the first step to preventing disease and catching cancer early.

Suggested tests

I commonly get questions about what type of screening is best, as well as what the risk factors are for the extra radiation exposure from the imaging studies. Overall, the impact of the radiation tends to equal the same amount of radiation you would get from taking a flight from Los Angeles to New York (about 6.5 hours). The benefits of screening outweigh the risks at this time. Although, I'm always keeping my eye out for updated technologies such as blood tests and thermograms that might rival the accuracy of the radiation-producing images, the technology is still evolving and improving. At this time, I still recommend traditional imaging to my patients.

In addition to screening, there are certain blood tests that I recommend to monitor cancer risk. These tests move beyond typical tumor markers and into factors that might trigger tumor growth such as inflammation, blood sugar regulation, angiogenesis, hormones and growth factors, and immune function. Don't worry about all the terms right now. As I've mentioned, you may be feeling overwhelmed right now. This is simply a starting point for monitoring your health.

One of the benefits of getting this information from lab tests is that it can help you and your healthcare teams individualize treatments. The tendency I see in my office is to take *everything* you have read about online, and apply it to your own treatment plan. The downside is that you are likely applying a lot of 'cancer prevention' tools that you don't need. I prefer to focus on the individual's health and monitor changes through lab work.

A basic cancer prevention panel could include:

- CBC (complete blood count), which provides basic red and white blood cell information

- CMP (comprehensive metabolic panel), which lets you know how your kidneys and liver are functioning

- Thyroid panel, comprising TSH, free T3, and free T4

- Vitamin D, 25-hydroxy

- Cholesterol panel

- Fasting insulin

- HbA1c (hemaglobin A1c)

For women, consider occasional monitoring of your hormones:

- Total estrogen

- Estrone

- Estradiol

- DHEA-S

- Progesterone

- Testosterone

For men, consider monitoring:

- PSA

- Testosterone

- DHEA-S

For people with active cancer, I often recommend adding angiogenesis labs:

- VEGF (vascular endothelial growth factor)

- D-dimer

- Ceruloplasmin

- Copper

- Zinc

I might also recommend labs that track inflammation:

- Interleukin-6

- High sensitivity C-reactive protein

- Ferritin

Sometimes, we look at cancer growth factors such as:

- IGF-1 (insulin-like growth factor 1)

Occasionally, we will also look at immune system

balance through labs like:

- Natural killer cell response

- Viral titers

- Stool samples

- Microbiome samples

If you have significant environmental toxin exposure through your living situation, childhood, or occupation, I would also seek:

- Solvent panel

- Heavy metal panel

If you are under a lot of stress, suffer with insomnia, or are tired all the time, I suggest taking a look at:

- AM and PM cortisol

- Viral titers

Blood sugar management testing

Understanding how your body is managing sugar is an important piece of reducing cancer risk or risk of recurrence. A test often overlooked by many doctors is fasting insulin levels. Most offices look at fasting glucose by itself, but fail to take into account the role of insulin. Insulin is important because it is a hormone that regulates the amount of sugar in your blood, and helps sugar get to important tissues like your brain and muscles. Having elevated insulin levels is often the "pre-diabetes" state of sugar management. This is particularly important in cancer care because serum insulin, maybe even more directly than glucose, can be traced to tumor growth and risk of recurrence. You can get simple blood tests to see how your body is processing sugar and managing insulin.

Another blood test often overlooked that is related to insulin and glucose is insulin-like growth factor 1 (IGF-1). IGF-1 has been linked to growth of colon, breast, prostate, and pancreatic cancer. It is a cancer growth factor stimulated by insulin. When people say "sugar feeds cancer", I like to think that it's not just circulating glucose that is feeding cancer, but more likely IGF-1, a downstream consequence of sugar that is actually encouraging cancer growth.

The good news is that with the use of diet, exercise, and naturopathic medicine you can help control your insulin response, lower IGF-1, and reduce your risk of cancer recurrence. Some natural therapies for improving blood sugar, insulin, and IGF-1 balance include: berberine, fish oil, lycopene, green tea, and alpha lipoic acid just to name a few.

Inflammation testing

Inflammation is another one of the potential growth factors for cancer cells, and so it's well worth looking into testing in this area, especially given the emerging natural therapies. In testing for inflammation, we can look at more general inflammatory markers like C-reactive protein, or more specific inflammatory cytokines that directly stimulate cancer cell growth, such as interleukin-6 (IL-6). Elevated IL-6 has been associated with tumors that are resistant to treatment and increased tumor growth.

While there are no drugs on the market at this time for your medical oncologist to offer to lower IL-6, many natural extracts have been studied and found to have the potential to lower IL-6. Using integrative and naturopathic oncology in this area is interesting. Some natural therapies that have been studied for reducing IL-6 in the local tumor environment are curcumin, green tea, resveratrol, coptis, berberine, plant isoflavones, melatonin, and fish oil. This is an exciting area of more study since reducing IL-6 might help improve the efficacy of all cancer treatments.

Angiogenesis testing

Angiogenesis is the building of small microvessels in the body. These microvessels carry oxygen and nutrients to all tissues in your body. Cancer cells are particularly effective at creating extra microvessels. This is one of the ways they horde glucose and growth factors, causing them to multiply. To see if angiogenesis is contributing to your cancer risk or tumor growth, you can look at several nutrients and growth factors.

The growth factor that directly stimulates blood vessel growth is called vascular endothelial growth factor (VEGF). Certain conditions such as surgery and injury naturally increase VEGF for healing. During cancer growth, elevated VEGF is linked to a tumor that uses angiogenesis to grow. Some tumor types are more likely to use VEGF to its advantage than others. For example, kidney cancer is especially apt at doing so.

VEGF can be targeted by certain immunotherapies and chemotherapies. VEGF can also be targeted by natural therapies, in particular adding in dietary intakes of berries, green tea, fish oil, ginger, ginseng, wormwood, magnolia, mistletoe, skullcap, and curcumin.

I also like to look at copper levels in the blood because copper can stimulate VEGF. By balancing zinc and copper levels, we might be able to block angiogenesis and cancer growth. In fact, one therapy that is being investigated for stopping tumor growth is a copper-chelating agent. Zinc is a natural copper chelator, but it is not safe to take high levels of zinc without getting your copper and zinc levels tested first.

Hormones

You might already know that estrogen is linked to breast cancer growth. But did you know that estrogen is also linked to melanoma, lung cancer, and colon cancer to name just a few? Other hormones that have been linked to tumor growth include testosterone, DHEA, IGF-1, and human growth hormone (HGH), among others.

Certain natural therapies can balance out hormones identified in the blood stream as being elevated. Sometimes this includes adding mushrooms and flaxseeds to the diet. Other times a more concentrated approach with supplements from broccoli extracts such as DIM, or herbs like saw palmetto, or the nutrient calcium-d-glucarate might be in order. Some lifestyle factors that help balance hormones include exercising regularly, eating plenty of vegetables, drinking rBGH-free dairy, and reducing meat intake.

Immune function

Often I have patients saying to me that their main reason for being in my office is to "boost their immune system." The downside of boosting the immune system is that cancer uses an overactive immune system to its advantage just as much as it uses an underactive immune system. In my work, I like to talk about *balancing* the immune system. This means we need to know what your current immune status is to be able to tell if we need to boost or downregulate your immune system.

The tests I use to look at immune function can include natural killer cell testing and activity, vitamin D levels, CBC, ANA, autoimmune antibodies, and viral titers. Don't worry about all these initials! It's all just information to talk over with your healthcare team to help balance immune function. Depending on your lab results and the state of your immune system, you could use wheat germ extract, probiotics, berry extracts, ashwagandha, astragalus, mushrooms, and so many more dietary supplements individualized to your situation.

Genes and cancer

Genes and cancer have so many medical and science terms. I promise to help make this easy to understand and useable as possible. Let's take a deep breath together, and dive in.

Did you know that only 5% of people with cancer have a specific genetic mutation associated with cancer? And even if you're not in that 5%, that doesn't mean your genes don't matter! There is a new field of medicine called epigenetics, which as it turns out, could play a huge role in where cancer growth all starts.

First of all, if you have a strong family history of breast cancer, ovarian cancer, male breast cancer, or estrogen-receptor-negative breast cancer, it is a good idea to have genetic testing for the gene associated with breast cancer. The genes associated with breast and ovarian cancer are BRCA1 and BRCA2. Other cancers linked to BRCA1 and BRCA2 are prostate, uterine, cervical, and pancreatic cancer.

Another time to look at genetic risk for cancer is when you have a family history of Lynch syndrome cancers. The cancers associated with Lynch syndrome include colorectal, pancreatic, renal, endometrial, bile duct, stomach, and brain cancer. If a family member has more than one of these tumor types, or multiple family members on the same side of your family have had these types of tumors, it is a good idea to have your risk of Lynch syndrome evaluated by your doctor.

If you do have one of these types of familial cancer syndromes, it is not a death sentence. It does not mean you will 100% get cancer, even though your risk might be higher. Some strategies that have been shown in research studies to reduce the risk of a genetic cancer expressing itself include: eating vegetables, taking curcumin, exercise, and having adequate folate levels. None of these strategies is particularly invasive.

If you don't have one of these types of familial cancer syndromes, genetics can still influence your cancer risk. As mentioned above, there are epigenetics that are also associated with cancer risk. Epigenetics is defined as "the study of changes in organisms caused by modification of gene expression rather than alteration of the genetic code itself." This means genes are not fixed, but their expression may actually change.

Not only can your epigenetics change, but your epigenetic markers can be passed down through at least four generations. That means your epigenetics reflect your great-great-great-grandparents' genetics and every generation in between. We talk more about the accumulation of toxins over these generations in Chapter

5: Detox. So stay tuned for more info here!

Currently, we have over 80,000 chemicals on the market that influence these genes and could increase cancer risk. These chemical exposures as well as diet and lifestyle can lead to epigenetic changes and SNPs (pronounced *snips*). A SNP is a genetic variation found between genes. The simplest way to think of a SNP is to think of it as a typo in the DNA. For the most part, our body can overcome these SNPs, but put in the right (or wrong) environment, these SNPs can be associated with cancer growth.

Still keeping up? I promise we're almost done talking gene types!

The importance of knowing this information about your own genome is to help support optimal functioning of your genes. You can't reverse the SNPs, but you might be able to optimize function using supplements, diet choices, and lifestyle practices. Some of the genes influenced by epigenetics and SNPs, and that have been associated with an increased risk of cancer growth include: MTHFR, COMT, VDR, GSTM1, GSTP1, GSTT1, CYP1B1, CYP1A1, CYP1A2, CYP2D6, CYP3A4.

The science of using genetic information to optimize health and prevent cancer growth is still emerging. I prefer that the people I work with be on the cutting edge of medical technology and personal health information, so I include it here. It is important, especially in doing all that you can in picking the correct supplements, lifestyle changes, medications, and conventional cancer treatments. You can learn your SNPs through 23andMe or a variety of tests coming to market, like those offered to my patients in my office.

In addition to epigenetic, SNP, and whole body genetic information, the practice of oncology is moving towards understanding the genetic environment of the tumor. The tumor genetic environment can be different from person to person. With this individualized treatment comes individualized therapies from immunotherapies and chemotherapy to natural therapies. Customized genetic information about the tumor can be done with pathology samples from surgery and biopsies.

Occasionally, this specific genetic information can also be determined by capturing tumor cells circulating in the blood stream, also known as CTCs. This procedure is known as a "liquid biopsy." While this is a new technology, I highly recommend that my patients understand their tumor as in-depth as possible, because if you don't know your unique tumor qualities, how can you treat it uniquely?

The more you know about your body before, during, and after cancer, the more specific a treatment plan can be developed. In my opinion, individualizing your treatment is the secret sauce to more effective use of natural therapies. Knowing your individual risk factors is an imperative part of living a *Cancer Proof* lifestyle.

Yet knowledge alone is not enough to make real change happen. In the coming chapters, we start to look at how you can take meaningful action on your health.

CHAPTER 2:
GET MOVING

❋ — ❋ — ❋

You may know that moving your body is one key element of reducing your cancer risk, but exercise is a vast and loaded topic. So where do you start?

In this chapter, we'll look at:

- what sitting still is doing to your body and cancer growth

- how exercise prevents cancer cells growing and spreading

- the type of exercise that's best

- gentle movement solution.

Shaking up your sedentary lifestyle

Have you heard the phrase "sitting is the new smoking"? Researchers are calling sitting as bad as smoking for risk of and mortality from disease. This led to the rise of stand-up desks. However, there's conflicting information on whether or not standing is any better than sitting, because standing still has its own risk factors.

What we do know for definite is that being sedentary has negative impacts on our health.

One of the running jokes in my family is how TV-watching has become our new hobby. A little binge-watching of a TV show to get through a whole season, and somehow it feels like you accomplished something. Unfortunately, all that we really accomplished is sitting on the couch for at least 24 hours! And all jokes aside, this type of hobby is concerning.

Any time we spend sitting beyond two hours, we increase our risk of multiple types of cancer in a statistically significantly manner. If you break that up — so for example, let's say you only watch two episodes in a row and then get up and walk around, and then go back to bingeing for another two episodes — that break of movement actually provides some relief in that increased risk.

In addition, if you watch more than 14 hours of TV per week, you increase your risk of endometrial and colorectal cancer statistically significantly. That's two hours per day. As we take a moment and think about your life, how many DVR sessions or Netflix episodes is that? And it's not just endometrial and colon cancer risk that increase either. Two hours per day statistically significantly increases your risk of all types of cancer. Increase the TV-watching to 21 hours per week and the risk with colorectal cancer becomes worse still as it increases the risk of dying of the disease.

To make this more practical, let's do some TV-watching math. If you're getting home from work around 6:00 PM, maybe cooking dinner and doing household chores until 7:00 PM, then what are you doing the rest of the night until you go to sleep at 10:00 PM? Generally, we are sitting down and having screen time. That's why they say that sitting is the new smoking.

It's not just screen time that impacts our health. Any time that you sit for longer than two hours, you're greatly increasing your risk of cancer. It doesn't matter if you are sitting to watch TV, read a book, play a video game, or are on your computer. Just sitting for two hours increases cancer risk. I don't know about what your work day looks like, but I can easily go two hours of sitting still in front of my computer at work. And walking that 20 steps to get a drink or pick something up off the printer really doesn't count as physical activity!

How much is enough?

Given that this sedentary lifestyle is doing us no good, let's shift our attention to movement — one of the top lifestyle changes you can make to reduce cancer risk and help your body recover from cancer. Sounds easy enough, but what type of exercise should you be doing? Group exercise? Interval training? Walking?

At this time, research about exercise and cancer risk or risk of recurrence focuses on the number of minutes you exercise per week. And that magic number for exercise is 150 minutes per week. You can break up the 150 minutes between 5 days or 7 days. So, if you are exercising 5 days a week that's only 30 minutes a day. Alternatively, you could exercise for 150 minutes in a 'weekend warrior' kind of way, but there are additional protective benefits of exercising daily. A weekend warrior is anybody who is exercising greater than 75 minutes, and doing this twice per week. Even more committed is the weekend warrior who exercises for 150 minutes all at once! That could be a long hike, a run, a bike ride, any type of physical activity for a 150-minute stretch.

The takeaway message here is to get movement into your life. You have to ask yourself, what makes exercise a little bit easier to handle? Would it be easier to do 20 to 30 minutes a day, or 150 minutes in one or two days? Whatever your answer, let's get started.

Once you decide how you are going to get 150 minutes of exercise per week, the next step is accountability. What the research studies find is that when we are paying for accountability and have someone helping us, whether that's a physical therapist or a personal trainer, our compliance increases, outcomes improve, and overall it helps reduce risk of cancer and cancer recurrence. So here's your prescription: go ahead and find someone to help you start your commitment to movement. If you can't hire a professional to help keep you accountable to your movement goals, you could use a fitness tracker. According to researchers, fitness trackers can also be effective in helping you stay committed to your fitness goals.

There are several ways exercise impacts cancer cell growth specifically. Some of the benefits of exercise include:

- reducing metabolic syndrome

- reducing IGF-1, a cancer growth factor, especially in women with breast cancer, and supporting insulin

- improving vitamin D levels in your blood, a nutrient that is linked to reduced cancer risk and improved response to cancer treatment

- helping with DNA repair, an important step in protecting healthy cells and avoiding cancer cells

- reducing the cancer growth messenger and inflammatory response interleukin-6

- increasing bone density

- reducing death from cancer

- reducing 'chemo brain' when you exercise outside

- increasing natural killer cells, which are important in destroying tumors.

Even during cancer treatments, exercise can help by:

- reversing weight gain, blood sugar changes, and stress experienced due to cancer treatments

- improving sleep

- increasing energy levels

- reducing fatigue

- improving pain from treatments

- improving sexuality and intimacy, particularly after treatment for breast and prostate cancer.

Emotional benefits of exercise

Exercise can positively impact a lot more than just the physical aspects of wellbeing. Researchers found that one of the other benefits of exercise in all cancer types is improving self-image. Sometimes, after being diagnosed with cancer and going through cancer treatments, it can be a time of disconnection from the body. Other times, people may feel "betrayed" by their physical body for expressing a cancer in the first place. And I've also seen patients so wiped out after cancer treatment that they don't even know how to become physically active again.

If this sounds like you, whether you have been diagnosed with cancer or not, it's important to know that exercise can help you reconnect with your body. Starting an exercise and movement routine gives you a better sense of self. Once you can see yourself as physically strong again, this strength and empowerment can help you feel prepared to overcome your tumor.

As a healer and physician, I have seen the power of physical exercise to push people into a greater sense of survivorship. After having cancer in remission for several years, one of my patients joined me on a retreat to Maui, and experienced a huge mindset shift and reconnection with her physical body after a hike in Iao Valley.

This hike was particularly strenuous as we moved through a beautiful section of tropical rainforest. We were being led on our hike by a Mauian native who was not going to accept any self-perceived limitations as a barrier to crossing this sacred land. During the hike, many members of our party confronted fears; some even shed a few tears. Nobody was in physical danger, but we were bumping up against a lot of "upper limit" issues.

When we concluded our hike, one of the participants looked at me and said, "I forgot I was that strong." She had experienced a reconnection to her body and strength, which led to a breakthrough realization that she had fully come out the other side of her cancer diagnosis. In the years since, this retreat-goer has pointed back to our Maui hike as the moment she realized that she was done with cancer and able to live her life again... without limitations.

Potential dangers of exercise

One concern you may have heard about exercise is that

high-intensity exercise can cause oxidative stress and damage. In fact, I used to be concerned about this for my patients too. Which caused me to recommend keeping exercise to light or moderate activity. I didn't want to increase the oxidative stress through exercise.

Oxidative stress is the damage that can cause DNA changes. The harder we work out and the more intense we go, the more lactic acid we produce in our body; the more lactic acid, the more oxidative damage. Now, that is not such a bad thing in somebody who's healthy, but for someone who's going through cancer treatment, a high level of oxidative stress and oxidative damage is already occurring through their cancer treatments.

More recently, I've come across the good news. The research shows that intense exercise does not, in fact, increase oxidative damage in people who are actively going through cancer treatments. This exciting information means I encourage all different types of exercise without the fear of that exercise causing further oxidative stress. So with that in mind…

What type of exercise should you do?

There are so many ways to get yourself moving more in your life. Like all things, this should be individualized to you, your preferences, and your health status. Personally, I prefer little dance breaks in my office, kitchen, and just about anywhere else! What's important is that we are moving, it's fun, and it's something we can do regularly.

Remember, we are always individualizing.

Let's talk about the different types of exercise available to you.

Low-intensity exercise

Low-intensity exercise provides many health benefits, including one of the great benefits in cancer care: improving energy. It also reduces anemia, which can be important for anyone with cancer. Sometimes getting red blood cell counts back up during or after treatment, and getting platelets to normalize and stabilize, can be a challenge — even with the best natural therapies. Low-intensity exercise improves anemia scores, and should definitely be considered.

Some types of low-intensity movement include walking, gentle yoga, ballroom dancing, and tai chi.

Ballroom dancing has been studied in cancer survivors, and shown to improve quality of life and overall wellness factors.

Yoga has been found to be as beneficial as other types of exercise for people with cancer, cancer survivors, and in cancer prevention. Not all yoga is low intensity, though, so be mindful of your heart rate monitor to make sure you are doing the right yoga for where you're at in your health.

One of the benefits of yoga is that it improves balance.

We often see muscle weakness and lack of balance control, particularly in patients undergoing cancer treatments that lead to oxidative stress to the brain from radiation and other types of interventions.

As a yoga teacher, this type of movement has a special place in my heart. If you'd like to give yoga a try, check out this video practice that I put together especially for you at: http://drheatherpaulson.com/bookresources/

High-intensity exercise

High-intensity training — just the name of it can sound intimidating. If you hear this and break into a cold sweat over the idea of joining a bootcamp or crossfit situation, have no fear! When I'm talking to patients about exercise, I'm always reassuring them, "You don't have to go to bootcamp. I swear. You don't have to go to bootcamp."

However, doing more high-intensity exercise does help increase overall strength, improve body mass index, and reduce the percentage of fat that we carry. High-intensity exercise has also been shown to improve body image more than low-intensity exercise.

While reading the research studies, one of the interesting points that stood out to me when compared to low-intensity exercise is that cancer survivors doing high-intensity exercise had:

- a greater *sense* of self

- improved *sense* of strength

- a better *sense* of being able to overcome their disease

- reduced fear of dying from cancer.

Beyond the physical components of high-intensity exercise, the emotional benefits can be a huge piece in feeling like you can get your life back after cancer. If you're looking to prevent cancer, having strength and a sense of self will help you make the choices that benefit your overall health and wellness.

Why does high-intensity exercise work for blocking cancer growth and metastasis? Now, this is where it gets really interesting when it comes to preventing cancer growth. Exercise researchers have found that with high-intensity exercise, there's an increase in *shear force* going through the blood vessels. Shear force is a physics term that simply means that when fluid is flowing through a tube (like blood traveling through an artery), there is friction between the fluid and the tube. This friction is defined as shear stress or shear force. When we have circulating tumor cells in the blood stream, increasing shear force in a blood vessel actually causes apoptosis, or cell death, of the cancer cells.

Studies have found that 90% of circulating tumor cells are completely gone within four hours of high-intensity exercise. Ninety percent! That is a huge number and highly impactful for your health. In addition to the original 90% of circulating cancer cells going into apoptosis within a few hours of high-intensity exercise, there are more benefits! The cool thing is that the 10% of circulating tumor cells still left also die within 16 to 24 hours of that episode of high-intensity exercise! Completely undetectable. If we had a drug that could impact 100% of circulating tumor cells, that would be a phenomenal drug, wouldn't you agree? But we don't have a drug or supplement that has that level of efficacy. All we have is exercise.

Some examples of high-intensity exercise according to the World Health Organization include running, walking briskly up a hill, fast cycling, aerobics, fast swimming, and competitive sports.

One particularly interesting form of high-intensity exercise is triathlon. There have been studies showing that triathletes gain positive benefits from doing a triathlon or training for one after cancer treatments. Training for a triathlon improves long-term health, so even long after a single triathlon event is done, the cancer patients who trained were more likely to stick with the diet and lifestyle changes than cancer patients who didn't.

Training for a half marathon was one of the ways my husband Phil conquered cancer. Phil is a lymphoma survivor. Six months after he finished nine months of chemotherapy, we ran a half marathon together. I was in my first year of medical school, and I thought it was absolutely crazy for him to do a half marathon right after chemo. I kept asking, "Why are we doing this? This is crazy. You're so depleted. You should not be running a half marathon."

What I learned from that experience and what the studies support is that Phil felt more connected to his body during the training sessions than he had in a long, long time, and certainly since before his lymphoma. During cancer treatment, he had felt depleted, abnormal, and unhealthy. He was kind of down about himself to be honest. He found that doing a half marathon helped him feel super strong and reconnected to his own strength. It was amazing to see the change in him after the experience.

Thinking about that time in our life gets me a little choked up, because after completing that half marathon, there was this immediate shift, like, "Okay, I can go back to a normal life. I'm healthy. I'm not a cancer survivor. I'm a healthy person. I have what it takes to truly have long-term survival."

Phil would probably say it a little differently, but that's me interpreting what I witnessed!

Weight-lifting

Another way to increase exercise intensity is with weights. Weight-lifting has its own benefits for reducing lymphedema in women who underwent surgery for breast cancer. Early on in my cancer career, I advised my patients to avoid weight-lifting because I was concerned that it might increase edema or cause strain in the extremities. However, the studies now support weight-lifting for improving extremity muscle strength, reducing risk of lymphedema, progression of lymphedema, and even reversing lymphedema for patients who already had it present.

Weight-lifting happens in both concentric and eccentric directions. Concentric is any time we are shortening a muscle and eccentric is any time a muscle lengthens. Some early animal studies are looking at whether a certain type of muscle movement is more protective against cancer growth than another. Early studies are pointing towards eccentric exercise being more protective.

But how do you only lengthen your muscles? An easy way to do this is through adaptive resistance exercise or ARX. This is an exercise machine based on a computer system that tracks the amount of resistance or force you exert when you pull or push. The computer matches your force, so you are essentially pulling or pushing against your own strength. I was first introduced to ARX by listening to Dave Asprey's Bulletproof podcast.

One of the reasons I recommend ARX to my patients is because, since you are only working against your own strength, it starts exactly where you are. This machine can be used to be protective against joint space that is at risk of injury. It can also track exactly how much strength you are building in an objective way. At this time, there's only a couple centers throughout the U.S. that have these machines, but if you can get to one, I highly recommend it.

Personalizing your plan

Now comes the important piece: personalizing movement for your body. I have laid out several options from low intensity to high intensity, from group exercise to running by yourself. Studies comparing high-intensity to low-intensity exercise found no overall benefit in one type of exercise over another. That means, whatever you choose, you will have some health benefits. To help you personalize your activity plan, I recommend reflecting on the following:

I am not active because...

I am or want to be active because...

When I exercise or am active, I feel...

This week, I commit to...

You can do this! Remember to ask for help if you need it. Have your doctor refer you to physical therapy if needed. Whatever you do, make sure you can start exercising.

Julie's story

"How would you like to take a hike to the Iao Valley with

Kahu Kamuela?" asked Dr. Paulson. We had just begun our Cancer Survivors Retreat, which Rev. Kamuela had started off so beautifully, welcoming us to Maui and blessing our stay with an opening ceremony featuring his two daughters performing authentic hula dancing for us. That sounded kinda dreamy, a hike in the Iao Valley. So, of course, I immediately said yes!

I was a couple of years out from my cancer diagnosis, feeling pretty fragile in body and spirit. Attending this retreat had been my goal all year and I wanted it to mark the beginning of my healing, my return to total health.

Wednesday morning came and off we went, arriving in such a wondrous place. A beautiful creek winding its way down between the giant line of green velvet mountains and a beckoning, a nicely paved trail leading us towards it. It was sweet, walking through the dense forest, listening to the sound of the water and Kahu explaining the history of the area. The battle his ancestors, the Maui natives, had fought with King Kamehameha.

And then the paving ended, but the trail did not. And so we walked on. Somewhere along the way we stopped and Kahu performed another ceremony, allowing us to enter this holy space respectfully. The trail began to climb a little thereafter. Kahu said he wanted to take us to the top, because there was something he wanted us to see and experience up there. No worries, we were not racing; we rested frequently and I was fine.

At some point, we stopped. This is where our trail would end and our trial would begin. Kahu pointed straight up. We were going to start climbing. Using exposed roots and rock crannies, we were going to climb. My first thought was: no way! Yet Kahu is a mountain of a man and I absolutely trusted him and Dr. Paulson. If worst came to worst, I figured he could just carry me, so up we went. Climbing higher and higher. If I looked up and saw where we were to go, it was too much, too overwhelming, and so I focused on just the next step, just the next few feet, where I would place my hands and feet as we slowly made our way up.

Finally, we came to a huge, fallen tree blocking our path. Kahu looked for a way around it in either direction. Alas, there was none and so, after a rest, we began our descent. Climbing down the way we had come. Somewhere along the way, I ended up in front, leading the group down. How did that happen? And as we made our way back to the trail and vehicle, that thought echoed so loudly in my head. "You are leading this group!!" I said it out loud. Where did fragile, disabled Julie go? I guess I left her somewhere along the climb up and I don't miss her.

Had I known what hiking the Iao Valley entailed, I would never have even tried it. I have had bad knees for a long, long time, way before the cancer. Combining that with the level of ability I thought I had, well, there would be no way I'd have thought I could manage such a trek. I would have stayed behind. I'm sure several others in the group would echo that sentiment. But we all went and we all made it up and down. No man left behind and everybody was just fine. Miraculous.

The hike was not on our itinerary. It was a gift to us from Rev. Kamuela. And what a gift it was, allowing me to reconnect with myself and to find everything I thought cancer had stolen.

Julie Kenkel

CHAPTER 3:
DISCOVER YOUR IDEAL DIET

❋—❋—❋

What should I eat to help treat my cancer? What food should I stay away from now that I have cancer? What can I include in my diet to help me stay cancer-free? These are easily the most common questions I get in my practice. And in this chapter we are going to tackle just that — food for a *Cancer Proof* life.

Here's what we'll go into:

- which cancer diet is best for you

- how to shift your diet

- what you should absolutely stay away from

- what to eat instead (recipes included!)

Simplifying your relationship with food

So often, what we feel we "should" eat and drink is defined by strict diet plans in books focused on weight loss or healing. When we think about food from a position of "should", our relationship with food gets defined by phrases like *I'm raw, I'm vegan, I'm paleo,*

I'm gluten-free and so on.

I've found that when my patients restrict themselves to these definitions of how we "should" eat and what we "should" eat, it doesn't allow for the uniqueness of each individual and what works for their body. It really doesn't need to be so prescriptive or so complicated.

When we step back and look at the nutrition research for diets that *prevent* disease, including cancer, the recommendations are pretty simple. Epidemiological studies support a diet that focuses on eating vegetables and whole grains for important nutrients, minerals, fats, and vitamins. It is also recommended to focus on proteins for amino acids. These proteins can come from animals or plants. The research studies are clear that avoiding saturated fats and maintaining a low red meat diet reduces cancer risk and risk of recurrence. As an extension to this, I would advise avoiding pork altogether, focusing animal proteins on fish and fowl.

Another area where the research is clear about increasing cancer risk and risk of recurrence has to do with your weight. A high body mass index (BMI) is a known risk factor for cancer recurrence. Even losing 10 pounds or 4.5 kilograms has been shown to reduce cancer risk dramatically.

If you've been diagnosed with cancer or tried to look into cancer-preventative diets you've probably gotten pretty confused or maybe just overwhelmed. The cancer diets on the internet can range from going vegan and completely letting go of all animal proteins to having a ketogenic diet that is mostly meat-based and strict on how many carbohydrates or vegetables you can take in. Between those two diets, there's got to be a middle ground. I want to help you take your cancer diet from confusion to clarity. To do that, we'll be looking at how eating got so complicated.

Food is something we need for survival, and yet it's become difficult to figure out what to eat, how to eat, and how to cook. Together, we are going to go through all of the most common cancer diet suggestions. I'll cover the myths and legends, and what the research says. Most importantly, by the end of this chapter, it will all be simplified so that you can make the right choices for your diet right now.

The most common diets I hear about from patients in my office are: paleo, ketogenic, vegan, and raw. Some other diets you might come across are macrobiotic and juicing. Want to know the shocking truth? I don't recommend *any* of these diets! Why? Let's take a walk through each diet and look at their benefits and downsides so you can make some clear choices going forward.

Paleo

The *paleo diet* is a way of eating that's focused on animal-based proteins. It's generally high in fat, high in vegetables and high in fruit. When practicing a more traditional paleo diet, you're avoiding grains, all processed foods, and dairy. According to the people who started the paleo diet, eating this way resembles what our ancestors would've eaten in the Neanderthal and Paleolithic periods.

Benefits:

A paleo diet removes refined foods, which is incredibly beneficial for reducing risk of cancer recurrence. It also decreases sugar intake, which I highly recommend doing, because this is beneficial in balancing blood glucose and blood insulin levels, and reducing some hormones that respond to blood glucose and insulin that may increase cancer cell growth.

By inhibiting grain intake, a paleo diet also reduces lectin intake. The intake of lectins can increase inflammation in some individuals.

Downsides:

If done incorrectly, a paleo diet can be high in arachidonic acid, which has been linked to increased cancer growth. By eating grass-fed and grass-finished meats and wild-caught fish, you will consume less arachidonic acid.

Depending on which fats you choose to consume in a paleo diet, it might be high in saturated fat which has been clearly linked to an increased cancer risk and an increased risk of recurrence.

By eliminating all grains, you may be eliminating some important B vitamins that are needed to reduce risk of recurrence. Some of these B vitamins have only been shown to be beneficial in reducing cancer risk when taken through diet and not supplements. So you can't supplement your way out of this one. Furthermore, some lectins in grains have been shown reduce tumor cell growth.

Ketogenic

The *ketogenic diet* works by having 75% of its calories from fat, 20% of calories from protein, and only 5% of calories from carbohydrates, which is equivalent to 20 to 60 grams of carbohydrates per day. To put this into perspective, if you look at the nutrition label on whatever type of bread you use, it will already be over that 20 to 60 grams per day threshold *in just one slice of toast*.

In cancer care, the ketogenic diet works by exploiting the difference between cancer cells and normal cells. When comparing cancer cells to normal cells, the main differences are the way they use glucose and oxidation. Cancer cells have a greater glucose metabolism and mitochondrial oxidative metabolism, which is thought to cause chronic metabolic oxidative stress by switching the body's fuel from glucose to ketones.

Benefits:

The benefits of a ketogenic diet include decreasing sugar intake. It has also been shown to reduce insulin response, which can stimulate insulin-like growth factor, a hormone that has been linked to cancer cell growth. This hormone is discussed in further detail in Chapter 1: Know Yourself. People on a ketogenic diet tend to have improved blood sugar maintenance.

Some interesting studies have been published, utilizing a ketogenic diet to treat glioblastomas, brain tumors. Research studies found the glioblastoma tumors responded to and shrunk when the patients were on a ketogenic diet.

Downsides:

Some of the risks of a ketogenic diet are pretty similar to the risks of being paleo, which again revolve around the fact that it can be high in arachidonic acid, which causes inflammation.

Likewise with paleo, the high fat diet may increase cancer risk depending on the type of fat focused on. The ketogenic diet has been shown to cause serum deficiencies in trace minerals such as selenium, copper, and zinc. If you are prone to hypoglycemia, a ketogenic diet can cause nausea and low glucose.

When switching from glucose metabolism for energy to ketone metabolism, the acute changes can cause lethargy, nausea, and vomiting. This is especially true if you have a tendency towards hypoglycemia, because a ketogenic diet can lead to low glucose.

Changing to a ketogenic diet can also cause stomach and gastrointestinal upset if you have a hard time digesting fats. One study identified an increase in cholesterol in participants who had been on the ketogenic diet for one year.

There is currently an investigation into what is being called the "reverse Warburg effect" in cancer cell growth. These studies show that some tumors can create energy from their own sugar source, not just exogenous (externally sourced) sugar. At this time, it is not clear which tumor types benefit from a ketogenic diet and which do not. This is an area where cancer research is currently expanding.

Vegetarian

A *vegetarian diet* focuses on plant-based proteins and is high in vegetables. It is different to a vegan diet because it can include animal products like butter, eggs, and honey. It seems like defining a vegetarian diet would be super simple. On the contrary! While in general a vegetarian diet means to focus on a plant-strong diet, a vegetarian diet can include occasional animal proteins and animal products like cheese and eggs. Some vegetarian diets even include fish and meat.

The many types of vegetarians tend to be broken into the following groups:

- Pescatarian, in which the person may eat eggs, fish, dairy, and occasional poultry and/or red meat.

- Lacto-Ovo Vegetarian, which allows milk and eggs.

- Lacto Vegetarian, which allows milk.

- Pollotarian, which allows chicken and turkey.

- Flexitarian, where the diet means being vegetarian as much as possible and adding in a couple of meat-based meals a couple of times a month.

Benefits:

A recent study showed that a pescatarian diet reduced the risk of colon cancer by more than 30%. Overall, vegetarians have about half the cancer risk of meat eaters.

Other benefits of a vegetarian diet, include removing foods high in saturated fats. When you take away animal-based proteins, you're taking away a lot of the sources of saturated fats in your diet. Choosing vegetarianism can also increase phytonutrients just like the vegan and raw diets, and it's protective against certain types of cancer.

Downsides:

Some risk of a vegetarian diet includes becoming a "carbotarian" — somebody who doesn't eat vegetables or beans on a vegetarian diet and who ends up eating a diet mostly comprised of carbohydrates like pasta, toast, and crackers. In fact, most vegetarian dishes in restaurants are designed for carbotarians. Ultimately, you want to be careful of overindulging in refined carbohydrates like pastas, breads, and cereals.

Another risk of a vegetarian diet is that vegetarians have been shown to have increased dental cavities. This may be due to the pH changes that happen in the mouth when you eat mostly grains and vegetables. This pH change allows bacteria linked to cavities to thrive.

A vegetarian diet, if done improperly, might create sugar imbalances. If you're not balancing out you carbohydrates, proteins and fats, you can have spikes in sugar and overall increases in sugar in your bloodstream, which could potentially cause some issues for reducing risk of cancer recurrence.

Vegan

A *vegan diet* focuses on a completely plant-based diet eliminating all animal products. While eating a vegan diet, you are getting your proteins from beans, legumes, nuts and seeds. You also eat vegetables, fruit, and grains without restrictions.

When you remove meat from your diet and are getting protein from beans, legumes, nuts and seeds, you need grains added into your diet so that you can have a complete amino acid profile. Amino acids are the building blocks for your muscles, skin, and cells in your body.

Benefits:

Being a vegan includes eating a diet that's rich in diverse plant phytochemicals. Plant phytochemicals are the chemicals in herbs, vegetables, and fruit that have been studied for reducing and blocking cancer cell growth.

Many spiritual traditions carry a belief that there are energetic or spiritual benefits in eating a vegan diet, allowing for the clearer flow of subtle healing energies. There might also be some spiritual benefits in not having animals as part of your energy system or part of your *karmic debt.*

Data from an Adventist Health Study showed that non-vegetarians had an increased risk of both colorectal and prostate cancer when compared to vegetarians. Other studies showed that vegan diets provided protection for overall cancer incidence, especially in female cancers.

Downsides:

One phrase we use in our house when we are eating junk food is: *it's vegan, so that means it's healthy... right?*

It can be pretty easy to eat a junk food vegan diet with vegan donuts, vegan candy bars, and vegan macaroni cheese. Even Oreos are vegan! So, just because something has the label "vegan" doesn't mean it's healthy!

A vegan diet can also cause several different nutrient depletions. The main nutrients depleted in a vegan diet are iron and vitamin B-12. It's also possible to become depleted in conditionally essential amino acids if you're not being careful. Some rarer nutrient deficiencies can include zinc and omega-3 fatty acids.

Macrobiotic

Next up is *the macrobiotic diet*, which focuses on eating foods that are in season. There are lots of greens, vegetables, beans and sea vegetables. For the most part, a macrobiotic diet avoids meat, processed or refined foods, juice, and anything that's stimulating, especially stimulating teas and hot spices.

On a daily basis, you would be eating whole cereal grains like pasta and noodles, flat bread and bread, vegetables, pickle beans and bean products, sea and water vegetables, vegetable oil, seasoning and condiments. A couple of times per week you might be adding seeds and nuts, natural sweets like dates and figs, fruits, and fish and seafood. Once a month, you can add fish, seafood, dairy, eggs and poultry, and meat. However, meat is optional and doesn't need to be used at all in a macrobiotic diet if you prefer to avoid it.

Benefits:

Healing centers that specialize in the macrobiotic diet have medically documented cancer cases reviewed by the National Cancer Institute in the United States for being an effective diet for reversing cancer growth in humans.

Downsides:

Some of the risks of a macrobiotic diet include potential deficiencies in vitamin B12. The macrobiotic diet also falls down in that it does not advocate for the use of supplements. In fact, people are discouraged from using supplements at all.

Some patients using a macrobiotic diet have reported that it can be difficult to find macrobiotic ingredients in the grocery store.

Raw

The *raw diet* is all about eating only foods that are kept at a low temperature; none of the food can go above 118°F or 48°C. Eating a raw diet requires you to stick to unprocessed foods, nuts and seeds, sprouted greens, vegetables, and fruit. When you're on a raw diet, it doesn't necessarily mean being vegetarian. You can eat raw fish, eggs, dairy, and meat as long as the food hasn't been cooked at a temperature above 118°F.

Benefits:

A raw diet might increase enzymes from food by keeping food at a low temperature. It is also very high in fiber, which has been known to reduce the risk of certain types of cancer, particularly colon cancer.

By definition, a raw diet is free of processed foods. That helps keep chemicals and sugars out of your diet.

Similar to a vegan diet, a raw diet is rich with phytochemicals that can help block tumor growth.

Downsides:

Some of the risks of a raw diet include getting low in nutrients like calcium and vitamin B-12, and also increasing your risk of food-borne illnesses and infections.

Another downside to the raw diet is that you might actually be missing out on some of the cancer-fighting phytochemicals that you can get from vegetables, such as lycopene and beta-carotene. The foods rich in lycopene and beta-carotene need to be cooked to improve the absorption of those two chemicals.

Juicing

Juicing is a popular one. You might have seen juice bars popping up in your local town or maybe the green juices available in your local grocery store. Juicing means having a liquid diet. Juices can be made from vegetables, fruit or a combination of the two. In a juicing diet, you're avoiding grains and processed foods as well as dairy.

Benefits:

Some of the benefits of juicing are that you could consume highly nutrient-dense juice, which is easily absorbed. There are tons and tons and tons of beneficial phytochemicals available to you when you eat this way.

Downsides:

A juicing diet can become low in protein, fiber, and caloric intake. There are also some risks with juicing in particular prescription drugs, so you want to make sure that you're not drinking any juices that inhibit your drugs from working.

Juicing can be high in sugar if you are not appropriately balancing some of the fruits with other ingredients. In fact, in some studies, juice was as bad for diabetes and blood sugar management as drinking soda.

Fasting

Fasting focuses on eating certain foods during certain hours of the day or not eating solid foods at all. You can do water fasting, juice fasting or intermittent fasting. When you choose this method, you're avoiding all solid foods, sugar and dairy.

Benefits:

Research studies are looking at utilizing a fasting diet for managing blood sugar and diabetes, as well as using it to reverse nerve pain or neuropathy. At the University of Southern California (USC), researchers are examining the possibilities of using fasting with chemotherapy to reduce chemotherapy side effects and possibly improve efficacy. It might also improve the immune system's ability to react to and get rid of cancer cells.

Intermittent fasting might also reduce risk of cancer risk. Women who fasted for 13 hours or more nightly had a reduced incidence of breast cancer recurrence.

Downsides:

Some of the risks of fasting include not taking in enough calories every day, becoming nutrient-deficient and risking doing harm to the liver and pancreas. Fasting should not be initiated without medical supervision.

What does it all mean?

Given that all these different diet options have their benefits and downsides, what can you do to make sure you're getting truly *Cancer Proof* nutrition? The good news is all diets just mentioned share some particular qualities that you can put into place in the way you eat right now.

These positive properties are:

- low in refined and processed foods

- limited sugar

- limited saturated fats

- high in phytonutrients and phytochemicals

- high in healthy fats.

Based on my clinical experience, these properties are where we should place our focus for shifting our diet, because they are the areas that can help create the biggest impact in reducing or preventing cancer cell growth.

Here's a bare minimum outline of where to start making shifts in your diet, according to Michael Pollan in his popular food manual *Food Rules*:

- don't eat anything with more than five ingredients

- don't eat anything that won't eventually rot

- shop on the perimeter of the store

- don't eat anything your great-grandmother wouldn't recognize as food

- avoid these ingredients: high fructose corn syrup, enriched flour, bleached flour, sugar, and hydrogenated oils.

So far, we've been focusing on simplifying diet for you. However, the relationship between sugar and cancer is a little more complex. Sugar has an indirect link to cancer growth and recurrence risk. It's important to learn how your body processes glucose, insulin, and IGF-1, because an elevated insulin level is a risk factor for cancer recurrence, as we covered in Chapter 1: Know Yourself.

Sugar isn't the only no-go zone, though. As Pollan's book mentions, it's well worth steering clear of hydrogenated oils, processed flours and high fructose corn syrup. This is where it starts to become less easy-to-follow and a bit more work figuring out what to eat, but don't give up now. To make it clearer, this is what I recommend to my patients:

Avoid	**Eat**
Processed flour: white flour, rice flour, soy flour, breads, bagels, muffins, buns, etc.	Whole grains: oatmeal that hasn't been processed, barley, spelt, flax, millet, quinoa, rice. For extra credit, add sprouted grains.
Animal protein: limit red meat to 18 ounces or less per week. This includes beef, lamb, and pork. Completely eliminate all processed meats.	Mixed proteins: incorporate a variety of proteins from plants and animals. Include sustainable fish, low heavy metal fish, beans,

Unsustainable or heavy-metal-rich fish.

seeds, and other occasional animal meats.

Omega 6 fats: highly present in factory-farmed meats, corn oil, cottonseed oil, soy oil.

Omega 3 fats: rich in wild-caught coldwater fish, nuts, flaxseeds, chia seeds, grape leaves, and walnuts.

Saturated fats: cheese, palm oil, dairy.

Unsaturated fats: olive oil, conjugated linoleic acid (CLA), avocados, nuts, cold-pressed vegetable oils.

Processed sugars: powdered or granulated sugars, juices.

Unprocessed sugars: whole fruit, honey, maple syrup, molasses.

Low fiber: less than 30 grams of fiber per day.

High fiber: 30 to 40 grams of fiber per day.

Alcohol: more than 3 servings per week.

Alcohol: 3 or fewer servings per week.

Toxins: pesticides, plastic, rBST, genetically modified (GMO), BPA

Non-toxic: organic, GMO-free, glass and stainless steel storage,

storage, antibiotics, unfiltered.

hormone-free, antibiotic-free, filtered.

There are also special phytochemicals that we focus on to help reduce cancer growth. No matter what type of diet you decide to implement, these beneficial nutrients and chemicals should be included somewhere.

Sulforaphanes

Sulforaphanes are sulfur-containing compounds that makes broccoli or Brussels sprouts give off that special smell in your kitchen after steaming. Sulforaphanes have been studied and found to be effective in reducing lung cancer risk in previous smokers. They've also been studied for reducing risk of breast cancer growth, liver issues, and positive benefits have been found including for melanoma and prostate cancer. Sulforaphanes can also increase glutathione in the liver, and help the body excrete and metabolize toxins and hormones.

Common sources:

garlic, onions, Brussels sprouts, spinach, kale, cabbage, bok choy, kohlrabi, broccoli, cauliflower

Carotenoids

Here's an area where we need to be wary. Beta-carotene as a supplement could be responsible for increasing cancer cell growth. What's interesting and might feel a little contradictory is that, in food form, beta-carotene actually reduces cancer cell growth. For the greatest benefit, you would want to focus on in your diet and not so much in capsule or pill form.

Beta-carotene is found in significant density in any fruits or vegetables that are orange in color, and also can be found in red or yellow fruits and vegetables.

Common sources:

carrots, orange peppers, squash, pumpkin, sweet potato, cantaloupe

Quercetin

A powerful cancer inhibitor, quercetin has been studied to inhibit cancer cell growth, reduce inflammation, and increase cancer cell death.

Common sources:

green tea, grapes, red raspberry, nectarine, broccoli, black tea, red wine, onions, garlic

Folate

Folate, like beta-carotene, is one of those nutrients that should be cautioned against when it comes to supplements. But when it comes to dietary intake, it's super protective for our genetic make-up, our DNA, to eat foods that are rich in folate. In fact, that's why folate is recommended to women who are pregnant; it helps with cell differentiation and cell replication particularly in the nervous system. There are a lot of foods to choose from in order to have a folate-rich diet.

Common sources:

leafy greens, asparagus, broccoli, citrus, beans and peas, avocados, okra, Brussels sprouts, nuts and seeds, beets, corn, celery, carrots and squash

Lycopene

Lycopene has been studied for reducing the risk of growth for breast cancer, prostate cancer, colon cancer and melanoma. Participants that had a greater lycopene concentration in their blood experienced the biggest benefits. One way to increase lycopene in your blood stream is to increase the frequency you eat lycopene-rich foods.

Lycopene is found in any foods that are red in color. One of the interesting things about lycopene is that it is better absorbed from cooked foods. For example, the longer you cook a tomato, the more lycopene is available for absorption. Foodstuffs like tomato paste, in which the tomatoes are cooked for hours and hours, are much higher in lycopene than cutting a fresh tomato.

Common sources:

tomatoes, strawberries, watermelon, red peppers

Flavonoids and anthocyanins

Flavonoids and anthocyanins are known for reducing inflammation and blood vessel growth in cancer cells. Without blood vessel growth, cancer cells can't have nutrients delivered into them. When we cut off the blood vessels, it's like cutting off the road that supplies the nutrients that increase cancer cell growth.

Common sources:

grapes, berries, tea, coffee, pomegranate

Beta-glucans

Beta-glucans may inhibit aromatase enzyme, which has been studied with breast cancer and prostate cancer. The aromatase enzyme helps convert estrogen and testosterone back and forth and it's one of the enzymes that's specifically targeted with aromatase inhibitors like Aromasin and Femara.

The other great aspect to beta-glucans is that they support immune function. They help your natural killer cells (or your immune cells that are responsible for tagging and eating up cancer) to function better. It takes as little as 16 ounces of mushrooms per week, or just a couple of handfuls.

Common sources:

mushrooms, oats, barley, yeast, seaweed

EGCg

EGCg (epigallocatechin gallate) may reduce circulating estrogens, block blood vessel growth of cancer cells, and help increase apoptosis or cancer cell death. It can also potentially reduce risk of cancer recurrence.

Common sources:

green tea, black tea, carob, cocoa, fuji apples, pecans, hazelnuts

Spices

Spices are a great source of anti-inflammatory cancer blockers. In the past, the majority of our medicine cabinet would be found on our spice rack.

Common sources:

ginger, turmeric, black pepper, chili pepper, oregano, rosemary

Fermented foods

Eating fermented foods helps create a healthy microbiome, which is the totality of microorganisms and their collective genetic material present in or on the human body. The microbiome and fermented foods stimulate the immune system to balance and regulate itself.

Common sources:

kefir, yogurt, kombucha, sauerkraut, kimchi

Individualizing your diet plan

The number one point to remember when it comes to dietary change is that nobody knows your body as well as you do and none of these generalized over-sweeping diet plans are individualized to you.

How do you know what diet makes you feel the best? Pay attention. Ask yourself how you feel after eating a meal. Energized? Clear? Light? Heavy? Brain fog? What are you craving? If you're tired or worn down, and reaching for caffeine to make it through your day, you might want to look at your diet to see if there's something that's making your body not feel its best. If you are energetic and feeling great, this is a great jumping-off point for you to incorporate particular foods that have been studied and shown to help reduce cancer cell growth.

Sometimes when we try to change our diet, it can bring up an emotional response or pattern. I want to make sure that your diet is supporting your health and wellbeing on multiple levels; not just your physical body, but also your emotional and energetic bodies. If you find diet changes bringing up harsh or disordered eating, please work with a support team that can help you find a healthy way to balance your food. At The Paulson Center, we use hypnotherapy and counseling to support patients in making diet changes.

Individualizing your diet plan is about the *how* to eat, not the *what* to eat. Focusing on the how allows us to check in and see the way food is affecting our body without being constrained by what we've been told to eat by a specific diet plan or book. Far too often, I see my patients focusing on the what to eat, and sacrifice their overall health and wellness because of it.

One story of a patient that was impacted by focusing on the *what* is Beth. She came into the office with a diagnosis of chronic lymphocytic leukemia. When she entered the office, she was malnourished, tired, and bloated. She was following a raw and juicing diet because she read that eating that type of food would cure her cancer. The problem was her disease had caused an enlarged spleen. In Chinese medicine, a large spleen causes retention of dampness. Raw foods are also very damp.

Although Beth was tired and having nausea, she was reluctant to give up raw foods and juices because she thought that eating that type of food was going to cure her cancer. In reality, she could get the same exact vegetables by blending soups instead of juice. As soon as she changed the *how* of what she was eating, Beth started to regain energy, be able to nourish herself, reduced spleen enlargement, and even normalized her blood counts.

In traditional healing systems such as Ayurveda and Traditional Chinese Medicine, you are guided in how to pick your food in a way that supports your individual and unique constitution. So, if eating vegetables, whole grains, and some animal-based proteins is the *what*, using traditional medicine systems can give insight into the *how* to eat for your body.

In Ayurvedic medicine, there are three types of people in the world as defined by their dosha. While your dosha can have subtle shifts over time, your main dosha tends to be defined at birth. The three doshas — Vata, Pitta, and Kapha — have a combination of five elements. These five elements combine to create everything we can see, touch, and feel in our physical existence. The five elements are space, air, fire, water, and earth. Taking these elements into account in your constitution, Ayurveda helps to guide you toward the right foods to balance your body.

Traditional Chinese Medicine also defines your type by the elements, with the additional categorization of damp or dry, yin or yang. This information is another great way of getting to know yourself so that you can make diet choices based on what feels right to you. The study of the elements, damp/dry, yin/yang are too detailed to go into in this chapter. I will say that in general a cancer diagnosis is one of damp retention in Chinese medicine. Occasionally, it can also be a diagnosis of yin deficiency.

Our acupuncturist at The Paulson Center has pulled

together some resources for you to learn more. Access them at: http://drheatherpaulson.com/bookresources/

Another way to personalize your diet is by looking at your genetic profile. Did you know that certain genes make it easier or harder for you to process proteins and carbohydrates? I recommend to my patients that they learn what type of metabolizer they are before deciding to go paleo or vegetarian. In our office, we use a test by Genetic Directions to help determine what type of diet is best for each individual.

Sample meals

Breakfast:

> Quinoa hot breakfast cereal with berries and coconut milk

> Turkey sausage with gluten-free toast and a cup of tea

> Smoothie with berries, milk alternative, hemp protein powder

Lunch:

Salad

Vegetable soup

Dinner:

> Grilled fish with freshly steamed vegetables

Bunless turkey burger with baked sweet potato wedges

Alternatively, try one of the cancer-preventing dinner menus below.

Cancer-preventing dinner menu #1

- Ginger turmeric coleslaw

- Mediterranean baked fish (with tomatoes)

- Grilled pineapple with raspberry sauce

Cancer-preventing dinner menu #2

- Thai soup with lemongrass and mushrooms

- Dairy-free green tea ice cream

Cancer-preventing dinner menu #3

- Tomato soup

- Garlicky steamed broccoli

- Cinnamon sweet potato dessert

Juice recipe

Simple juice with cruciferous veggies, beta-carotene, and spices

- ½ bunch of kale

- 1 cucumber

- 1 handful of sprouts

- 1 apple

- 1 lemon, to taste

- 2 carrots

- 1 handful of parsley

- ½ inch nub of turmeric

Cancer-preventing dinner recipes

Ginger Turmeric Coleslaw

- ½ cup of mayonnaise

- ¼ cup of cider vinegar

- 2 tbsp Dijon mustard

- 14-oz package of coleslaw mix

- ½ small red onion

- ½ tsp kosher salt

- ¼ tsp ground black pepper

- ½ tsp ground ginger

- 1 tsp turmeric

Directions:

In a large bowl, whisk together mayonnaise, vinegar, mustard, ginger, and turmeric. Add vegetable mix to the bowl and combine with sauce. Season to taste.

Mediterranean Baked Fish

- 2 tsp olive oil

- 1 large onion, sliced

- One 16-oz BPA-free can of whole tomatoes, drained (reserve juice)

- 1 bay leaf

- 2 garlic cloves

- 1 cup of water or broth

- ½ cup of the reserved tomato juice from canned tomatoes

- ¼ cup of lemon juice

- 1 tbsp freshly grated lemon or orange peel

- 1 tsp fennel seeds, crushed

- ½ tsp dried oregano, crushed

- ½ tsp dried thyme, crushed

- ½ tsp dried basil, crushed

- Black pepper, to taste

- 1 lb fish fillets

Directions:

Heat oil in a Teflon-free pan. Sauté onion over medium heat for five minutes or until onions turn golden. Add all remaining ingredients, except fish. Bring to a simmer. Cook for 30 minutes, uncovered. Put fish fillets in a 10 x 6-inch baking dish and cover with simmering sauce. Bake uncovered at 375°F for 15 minutes, or until fish is cooked through and flakes easily with a fork.

Grilled Pineapple with Raspberry Sauce

- 1 pineapple cut into ½-inch thick slices

- 1 tbsp coconut oil

- 1 tsp ground cinnamon

- 12 oz frozen raspberries, thawed (reserve liquid)

- 1 tbsp maple syrup

- 1 tsp vanilla extract

- raspberry liquid from the thawed raspberries

Directions for raspberry sauce:

Pour liquid from thawed raspberries into a blender with raspberries, maple syrup, and vanilla. Blend until just about smooth on low.

Directions for grilled pineapple:

Place pineapple slices in container with coconut oil and cinnamon. Shake until well coated. Heat grill or grill pan. Coat with additional coconut oil. Grill for three to four minutes on each side. Serve warm with raspberry sauce drizzled on top.

Thai Soup with Lemongrass

I don't think I can top this recipe from Williams-Sonoma.

Dairy-Free Green Tea Ice Cream

Make your own, or buy it from SoDelicious.

- 1 can of coconut cream
- 1 cup of unsweetened vanilla coconut milk
- 2 tbsp matcha green tea powder
- ¼ cup of pitted dates
- ¼ cup of maple syrup

Directions:

Place all ingredients into a blender and blend until mixed to a smoothie-like consistency. Transfer blended liquid to a glass container, chill in the fridge for two to three hours. Place chilled liquid into your ice cream maker, and churn per ice cream maker instructions.

Tomato Soup

- 1 tbsp extra virgin olive oil

- 3 garlic cloves, minced

- 1 tsp Italian mixed herbs (substitute thyme, oregano, rosemary or basil if needed)

- Two 28-oz BPA-free cans of crushed tomatoes

- 2 cups of water or broth

- 1 head of cauliflower, steamed

- ¼ cup of raw unsalted cashews or raw blanched slivered almonds

Directions:

Heat oil in a large saucepan over medium heat. Add garlic, herbs, and crushed red pepper (optional). Stir until fragrant (about 30 seconds). Add tomatoes, water/broth and cauliflower. Simmer for 10 minutes. Stir in nuts. Pass liquid through the blender, one or two cups at a time. Blend until smooth. Return to saucepan and warm. Salt to taste.

Garlicky Steamed Broccoli

- 1 head of fresh broccoli or 1 bag frozen broccoli

- 3 garlic cloves, chopped

- ½ cup of water

- Salt and pepper, to taste

Directions:

Chop broccoli. Add garlic and water to a medium sauce pan, bring to a simmer. Add broccoli and steam until broccoli is tender and bright green. Remove pan from heat and serve.

Cinnamon Sweet Potato Dessert

- 1 to 4 sweet potatoes

- Sprinkle of cinnamon

- Enough coconut oil to "butter" the sweet potatoes

Directions:

Heat oven to 400°F. Pierce each sweet potato several times with a fork. Place sweet potatoes on a lined baking sheet. Bake until tender, about 45 minutes. Cut each sweet potato in half. Apply coconut oil and sprinkle with cinnamon.

CHAPTER 4:
TRULY TAKE CARE OF YOURSELF

※—※—※

There used to be a saying pinned to the wall in my gym that really struck me. "You are your most valuable asset." This is so true. Without yourself, your health, your wellness, what else can be accomplished? It's time to treat yourself like you are your most valuable asset, because self-care is really about self-love.

In this chapter, we're talking about:

- why self-care is not optional

- tools to help your emotions

- all things rest

- setting up a support team.

Self-care is not optional

And this chapter is probably the one you feel most unlike reading. It sounds a whole lot less sexy than diet or lab tests, but in my opinion, it's the most important chapter in this book. No matter what you are doing to *Cancer Proof* your life, if you're always giving to others more than you are giving yourself, it will be depleting. I say this to you out of love. If you don't care for or love yourself, doing "all the right things" with diet, supplements, exercise, and detoxification will only get you so far toward your health goals.

I admit it. Self-care wasn't always at the top of my to-do list or something I would spend time going into detail with my patients. I come to you in this chapter as someone who's learning right along with you. After so many years of seeing patients have patterns of taking care of others over themselves, self-sacrificing their own health for someone else, being worried that they aren't being or doing enough, or just putting themselves on the bottom of the pile, then showing up in my office, it's time for me to say *enough is enough!* Self-care is a non-optional piece of everyone's care plan.

How do I justify spending all this time on taking care of myself? Is it selfish? Honestly, sometimes self-care makes me feel massively high maintenance! I could easily say, "My patients need me. There's phone calls and emails to return. There are prescriptions to call in. I just can't take care of myself right now." And I bet you could talk yourself out of self-care for similar reasons at home or at work. Based on my conversations with patients, it's likely you have put off self-care because you don't want to feel selfish or high maintenance, but no...

On the contrary to being selfish, I truly believe that

taking time to optimize health through self-care allows me to accomplish more than my peers in the long run. People often ask how I get so much done in a short amount of time, and my answer is always, "I rest and take care of myself. And I meditate." What could an hour of self-care or rest give you the power to do? Heal, connect, take care of others with more compassion, and create important work in the world — these are just a few of the benefits I have seen.

When I first started my self-care practices, I had to have a conversation with myself every time. It went a little something like this, "As a doctor treating people with cancer, I really need to show up as my best, most well-rested self. My patients deserve that kind of care. They don't want a doctor who's cranky, needs a nap, or seems burnt-out. Now, go take a nap."

Your family, friends, clients, and customers deserve you at your best too. Being at your best means being well-rested and well-nourished. So, if self-care starts feeling selfish, remember the other people who benefit from your self-care too. Usually, they're the same people who lead you to feel like you can't do self-care.

For instance, I could easily recite all the things my patients need me for, the work to be done, the phone calls to return, but when I'm honest about who that is truly serving, it puts me in the role of martyr, self-sacrificer, and hero. These are the flip side of being a nurturer, caregiver, and a person who loves and cares deeply for others. Be aware of how this is showing up for you in your life.

Real cancer patient's plea on social media:

"Ladies, I had another surgery (no tumor this time) but my gallbladder. Apparently the chemotherapy destroyed it. Seriously, it's not talked about enough how much other "stuff" comes with treating cancer. I was giving up and losing hope. Year and a half of pain, shaving my head (surprisingly painful and unpleasant) and walking around with electrodes on my head. But feeling better now and hopeful also.

It's incredible how physical health influences our mental state. I am normally so cheerful and happy by nature and I was almost getting depressed. Another reason to make self-care a priority!

My question is this: how do I make sure that I don't "have to get seriously sick again" to justify self-care? I know it is not the only reason for my illnesses. I don't blame myself entirely. But when my doctor examined me before they decided on surgery, she told me: 'How could you even function with so much pain and nausea? You must have felt terrible for a long time.' The answer is that I just sort of got used to it and thought it was laziness. I will be so grateful for tips!"

So often I hear things like this in my office, on social media, and in support groups. Does this sound familiar to you too?

Most of our lives we are focused on the needs of others. We spend our time nurturing our children, our relationships, and our work. But the time to pause and take care of ourselves is often missed. In my practice, self-care is defined as the time you put aside to take care of yourself. It's care by you and for you. It's important that self-care is done deliberately and intentionally. Self-care is an act in which we define what we need and take active steps to meet those needs. It is time to nurture yourself, take care of yourself, and treat yourself the same way you take care of and treat others.

I recommend that self-care be done without distractions, and without guilt. This is not a time to multi-task. Slowing down and taking care of yourself deserves your attention, 100%. So, with that in mind, here are the strategies I have found helpful for myself and my patients. I hope they are helpful for you.

- taking conscious breaks
- asking for help
- breathing deeply
- taking a bath
- resting
- take a class
- exercising
- listening to your favorite music
- having a facial
- getting some fresh air
- drinking a cup of nourishing tea

- washing your
  face

- getting a
  massage

Your self-care practice might change throughout the cancer journey. If you are in a space of cancer prevention, your self-care practices might focus on detoxification and reducing stress. Some of my favorite self-care practices in this category include: sensory deprivation or salt floats, meditation, sauna, and massage.

If you are actively undergoing treatment for cancer, your self-care might focus on rest, movement, or letting go of previous commitments. Some of my favorite self-care practices for this time of life are: saying no, gratitude journaling, facials, and napping.

If you are done with treatment and reducing risk of recurrence, your self-care might include ways to improve immune balance and reduce toxic treatment build-up. Some practices to consider include: massage, acupuncture, and IV nutrients.

Moving into a space of embracing self-care is a huge mindset shift! As I said, I don't come into this as the world's leading expert on self-care. With my own health challenges going on, I had to be put on bed rest for multiple weeks at a time several times throughout a single year before I could grasp the concept of self-care and integrate it into my routine. I was at risk of *working myself to death* (literally!) according to my hematologist.

EFT or tapping

Still resisting self-care practices? I suggest starting with some EFT and tapping on the issues that are keeping you from looking after yourself first. EFT or tapping uses the acupuncture meridian system to help release emotional programs and triggers.

Using a technique like EFT or tapping can help you release the stories you have been told or have been telling yourself around self-care. To come up with what to focus on while tapping, try looking at issues and emotions that arise if you aren't "busy" or "doing" or "achieving" or "taking care of others." Do you feel guilty asking someone else to make dinner one night? Do you have trouble justifying a much-needed sleep-in? Explore those.

You can find some standard EFT scripts for the day-to-day, but if you are looking for guidance to use EFT for your healing, I love the work of Brad Yates. His YouTube channel has many videos to follow along and explore this powerful healing technique. You can find his channel here: https://www.youtube.com/user/eftwizard

You may also choose to work with an individual EFT practitioner to help you create your own scripts and breakthroughs. If you are looking for a practitioner in your local area, try here: https://aametinternational.org

Appeal to your logic

If your brain keeps getting in the way of resting by saying you're "too busy for self-care", you might need to take a look at the research in the book *The Power of Rest: Why Sleep Alone Is Not Enough* by Matthew Edlund. In this book, the author presents several research studies that prove resting is an important piece of taking care of your health. Once I read all this compelling research literature, my logic brain had the info it needed to rationalize resting.

Schedule rest and self-care

If self-care gets squeezed out of your day-to-day life, it needs a permanent place in your calendar. When I was first incorporating self-care practices and rest into my routine, I had to start blocking off a time of rest on my schedule. I started by deliberately taking Saturday mornings off, forbidding myself to do anything work-related or anything that was for anyone else's needs. I would then fill that time with things that were nourishing to me, such as walking my dogs, lying on the couch watching a favorite TV show, going to breakfast with my husband, walking around an art show.

In addition to this, I schedule regular self-care maintenance appointments with my chiropractor, acupuncturist, massage therapist, float tank, etc. Once it's scheduled, I know I will do it. These appointments range from every week to once a month. But they are non-negotiables in my life.

Create a team of support

No one can do it alone. In fact, we are biologically wired to only survive in a group of support. When I first started doing self-care practices, I had to engage my loved ones and employees to help set boundaries around my time and life. In fact, I still actively engage them to help me stay on track to a burnout-free life. My boundaries around taking care of others are super fluid. Without the people who love me stepping in, listening to me verbally commit to the boundaries I'd like to create, then helping me implement them, I would still be sick.

My office staff have permission to suggest that I shut my computer, go home, or rest at lunch hour. My husband takes seriously protecting my time for rest during our weekends and vacations. A best friend will remind me to meditate when I get into go-go-go mode. Without these people helping me stick to my health goal of rest and self-care I know I would be far less successful.

Take a nap

During my early days of self-care, I would have to plan naptime. Just like a little kid, I would have to say to myself, "Come on Heather, it's time for your nap." There are so many reasons why napping is important. When I read the book *Take A Nap! Change Your Life* by Mark Ehrman and Sara Mednick, it truly was life-changing.

Located right in the front of the brain, there is an area called the prefrontal cortex. The prefrontal cortex is where our decision-making happens. When we're stressed out and tired, it's harder for us to engage the prefrontal cortex, meaning the brain can't function or make good decisions.

We've all experienced this situation: trying to solve a problem or find something and ending up completely defeated. The next morning, we wake up and there's the solution to the problem or the item we thought we'd lost right in front of us. That's an example of the prefrontal cortex operating optimally or sub-optimally.

Furthermore, while sleeping, the synapses in your brain (the areas of your brain that talk to each other) create new connections and you're able to come up with new solutions that you weren't able to come up with before you went to sleep. Pretty cool, right? This should be a little bit of fuel for you to overcome fatigue and exhaustion by resting. How would you rather go through life?

There are negative consequences if you don't rest, so this goes out to those who need to read this. If you don't rest, you have increased risk of cardiovascular disease, and your brain doesn't function well, which even shows up on brain scans.

If you are wondering about the best time to rest, researchers have answered this question. Napping in the middle of the day helps maintain peak cognitive performance, even in people who are otherwise sleep-deprived. Research also shows that napping in the middle of the day for as little as 20 minutes helps you maintain the same cognitive performance as someone who slept an entire 7 to 9 hours per night. So, if you are sleep-deprived, napping can be a solution for improving brain function.

Napping for 20 minutes can help you get through the rest of your day. Research studies looking at mid-day naps showed a 40% increase in creativity, including creative problem-solving. Companies like Google have nap pods for a reason! It improves productivity.

Not only that, but napping can help with blood sugar regulation, reduces blood pressure, improves cardiovascular health, and increases your happiness quotient.

Have I converted you into a napper yet? If not, then maybe I can convince you to rest instead. You don't have to take a nap to get benefits. You may be someone who feels groggy taking naps or naps may prevent you from performing your best. If this is the case, you can simply take a break and do something different. Play a musical instrument, take a walk, sit in meditation. Do something that brings you joy and is a natural break from everything else you're doing that day.

Nourish yourself

When you see the word 'nourish', does your mind automatically jump to food? Nourishment is a deep word that can mean feeding your mind, body, or spirit. It's so easy to forget to nourish ourselves inside and out, and that's part of what leads to burnout.

Some simple ways to nourish yourself can be drinking a cup of health-promoting tea, taking a nap, getting a smoothie or green juice, spending time with a uplifting friend or loved one, putting fresh sheets on your bed… It can be anything really, so experiment with what feels good for you. And remember to nourish yourself *every single day*.

Do less

My worldview was completely rocked when I heard Greg McKeown give a talk about his book *Essentialism*. In his book, he repeats the mantra, "Less but better," in relation to productivity and success.

The great part of doing less is that what you decide to focus on has 100% of your energy. This is an idea we are all too familiar with during cancer, where so much energy is spent focusing on doctor's appointments, treatments, and scans.

For me, practicing having one pointed focus brought a more zen-like state into our household during my husband's cancer treatments. All we focused on was treatment and being together enjoying the little moments of joy, like our new puppy. When we returned to "normal life" and started becoming distracted by all of the other pulls on our attention from friends, work, and other commitments, life became overwhelming again!

"Less but better" reminds us that we can take a stand and protect our precious time to do what we love. Not only can we leave some breathing room for precious time to be in the space of loved ones, but I have also noticed that when I take the less-but-better approach to my to-do list, I'm able to pick out the projects that will have the greatest impact on the people I'm serving, or the kind of life I want to live. Once that one project is done, we can go on to the next project that will heighten the meaning and joy in our lives.

Say no

It sounds so easy to say no, but so many people, including myself, struggle with it. In fact, some of my patients say that this is one of the reasons why they are grateful for cancer. It was the first time they felt like they had a good enough reason to say no to commitments. Saying no is one of the best self-care strategies that you can have.

When I read *Essentialism*, I was struck by the message, "When you say no, you're saying yes to something else." That also goes to say that when you are saying yes, you are saying no to something else. If you are saying yes to something that is not serving your health, doesn't light you up, or is a mediocre goal, you're saying no to yourself. You're saying no to everything that fills you up. You're saying no to committing to what you really want to do or the way you want life to be. You might be saying no to taking care of yourself because you're saying yes to taking care of somebody else.

Isn't it interesting when we flip the yes and the no? If you have a hard time saying no, imagine what you're saying yes to instead, and see how it becomes easier to turn down what doesn't fulfil you.

Create rituals

Your body is a sacred space. Many religions and spiritual practices remind us that the body is the temple which houses the spirit, the Soul, or God within us. Sometimes we forget the hollowness of this temple. We start to connect it to external rewards, impressions, and movement. Establishing daily rituals allows you to tune into your body, hearing what it truly needs.

A ritual is "a series of actions followed regularly." Creating your own rituals of self-care allows a certain rhythm to enter your life. With a rhythm comes a habit, and habits become our life… what we do without having to think about it. By providing a gentle rhythm throughout your day, steady like a beating drum, you allow your body to line up and stay connected to its best health, highest good, and divine influence.

When establishing a daily practice, keep in mind these questions:

Is this supporting my wellbeing physically, emotionally, and spiritually?

Is this in alignment with the seasonal cycles?

Is this in alignment with my current life cycle?

I like to think of daily rituals as a way to open and close my day. Morning rituals can be a time to reconnect with earth after being in dreamland. It can be a time to set your intention for the day and connect with your spiritual practice. Having a grounding practice in the morning can help you set a steady course for the rest of your day.

The evening time can be a time to reflect and release the activities of the day. As you disconnect from the people and places of the past day, you can reconnect with the inner stillness and peace within yourself. Evening is a great time to gently walk yourself into a quiet state so you can experience peaceful sleep.

Some suggestions for morning rituals include: mindfully drinking a cup of coffee or tea, sitting outside and listening to nature, a sun salutation yoga practice, earthing, dry-brushing your skin, oil pulling, meditation, prayer, taking a walk, being out in the sun, or anything else you can think of that will support your day.

Some suggestions for evening rituals include: journaling,

gratitude practices, gentle yoga, a cup of calming herbal tea, or anything that helps you release and unwind from the day.

You can also create rituals that happen less frequently than daily. You can have monthly or weekly self-care practices like: massage, facials, pedicures, crafting or other creative outlets, or anything else that brings you joy.

If some of these rituals sound interesting to you, but you're not sure where to start, we have handouts, videos, and resources as a jumping-off point on the *Cancer Proof* resource page:
http://drheatherpaulson.com/bookresources/

Go on a retreat

If you find it hard to take care of yourself during your day-to-day life, going on a retreat can be a great way to plunge into self-care and establish daily rituals that you can then implement at home. One idea is to put aside some time for yourself to have a little mini-retreat. If you can't travel to an exotic retreat location, you can schedule a retreat in your home town by putting one whole day or just an afternoon of self-care activities in the calendar.

To get the most out of a retreat, I definitely recommend getting into a new environment. A retreat allows you to focus on yourself without the guilt or the temptation of the to-do list. It gives you some time to escape the day-to-day, break old patterns, and set new rituals in place. Better yet, when you travel to a retreat, you can have someone else do all the planning for you.

Another benefit of a retreat is connecting to people who want to support you. Sometimes all we need to take care of ourselves is a community that is there to help us and cheer us on. If you're having a hard time finding that, a retreat allows you to connect to a group of like-minded people who are there to uplift you.

All of these fantastic benefits are reasons we offer retreats at The Paulson Center. To get on the retreat waitlist or to be the first to know when a new retreat opens, visit my site at:
http://drheatherpaulson.com/bookresources/

Notice the little things

I consider myself lucky to have had the opportunity to spend time with a patient, who I'll call Cher, because it reminded me of the joys of a beach bonfire. You see, Cher was diagnosed with breast cancer, and she used this as a jumping-off point to start living one of her dreams. Her dream was to visit places all over North America in an RV. When she came for her appointment, she arrived straight from the beach (a good six-hour drive!) where she'd just spent time camping with her family over the weekend.

I was speaking to Cher about the crackling fire, the roasting of marshmallows, and all the beauty that goes with spending time with loved ones gathered around a fire. This brought Cher to sharing with me one of the greatest gifts she feels cancer taught her. Cher told me how much she now appreciates *slowing down*. Before cancer, she would multi-task and worry constantly about what wasn't getting done. Now that she had slowed down, Cher noticed deeper connections to her loved ones and more time to take care of herself. She also found she was seeing the beauty in the little moments of everyday life. Even walking the dog had become more precious, as she was more present.

When have you felt the benefits of slowing down? In my own life, I have to make an effort to keep the pace of life slow every once in a while. If I don't, all of a sudden, a year has whizzed by in a blur of tasks and to-dos. I remember visiting family in the city and, while sitting outside a café with my husband, we couldn't help but notice how hurriedly people came in and out. It seemed everyone was missing the absolutely gorgeous California day, the scent of the freshly baked breads, and opportunities to smile and say thank you to other human beings.

Rushing pumps the stress hormone *cortisol* throughout the body. When we pump too much cortisol, we can have a hard time recovering from stress. Plus, we miss out on life. Time to ask yourself what you've been missing while rushing about!

Breath awareness

Your breath is a feedback system to let you know if you are in fight-or-flight mode or rest state. Holding your breath or breathing in a shallow pattern is linked to stress and fight-or-flight sympathetic state. Pay attention to your breath and see what kind of information you get back. The times when I start holding my breath are a sure indicator that I need slow down.

Taking a deep breath resets our parasympathetic nervous system, which is responsible for rest and relaxation. Think of your breath as the ultimate stress ctrl-alt-del button. When under stress, the body's natural response is short, shallow breathing. That is the sympathetic system taking over. The parasympathetic or relaxation system likes to have long deep breaths.

Having this awareness is a great self-care practice, because it means you can do something about it by introducing a conscious deep breath. Next time you feel stressed out, inhale for a count of 6, hold your breath at the top of the inhale for a count of 3, and exhale for a count of 6, hold your breath at the bottom of the exhale for a count of 3. In research studies, as little as 30 seconds of deep breathing has been shown to reset the parasympathetic nervous system. That means, after just a few repetitions of these inhales and exhales, your body chemistry is already shifting from stress and mess to calm and centered.

Now that you have some self-care strategies, what do you think you can commit to right now, today, or this week to show yourself some love and care?

CHAPTER 5:
DETOX YOUR ENVIRONMENT, HOME, AND CELLS

❋—❋—❋

O ne of the most common questions I get in my office (especially when someone is finishing up chemo or radiation) is: *Can I detox my body from these harmful chemicals?* So that's exactly what we're diving into in this chapter.

We'll cover:

- detoxification in seven areas

- identifying cancer-promoting chemicals in your home

- safety of detoxing with cancer

- how to cleanse (with more recipes coming up!)

What's the deal on detoxing?

So, we know that the chemicals you are exposed to in cancer treatment are for the benefit of killing off cancer cells. But what is it doing to your normal cells? And is there a way to remove some of these toxins from the body? These are all smart questions, because on the other side of this question of detoxification, patients are really asking: *What will happen if I remove some of these chemicals from my body? Is it safe to detox? If so, when?*

To show how much of a hot topic this is, I'll let you in on something. I don't just get this question from my cancer patients. Other doctors ask me about detox and cancer too. And they have been to medical school! So if you're reflecting on these questions, congratulations! You're ahead of the curve and super tuned in to your body.

Cleansing is an important part of cancer survivorship because we know from research studies that cancer growth can be attributed to several lifestyle factors including what we eat, what we drink and the type of environment that we live in. We've gone into the food and drink links to cancer already in Chapter 3: Discover Your Ideal Diet. Environmental links to cancer can include: pesticide exposure, solvents like paints and paint thinners, fragrances, cleaners, and countless ingredients and substances lurking in our homes. These can all contribute to cancer growth.

The good news is that for most of us a cleanse or detox is completely safe. In fact, we will go over some ways that you can do a detox or a cleanse with using ingredients found in the average kitchen cupboard. This detox can be super gentle without forcing anything to go through the intestines (no laxatives here!) or the liver. It has been specially designed to avoid any harsh "dumping" of chemicals or toxins from your body.

Why wouldn't you want that dumping? A lot of people think a detox is there to help you *force* nasties out of the body. However, your body will feel a lot better if you *support* the removal of toxins from the body instead. This detox is focused on giving your body the right tools to help get the junk out of your system, which allows you to remove just the right amount of toxins at just the right time.

What happens if you force it? Well, it's kind of like Lucy and Ethel in the chocolate factory. Eventually your body just can't keep up! You can get detox reactions like headaches, pain, and inflammation. And worse of all, your body puts those kicked up toxins back into storage. The phrase "no pain, no gain" just doesn't apply here. If you have any detox symptoms, it might be time to back off.

Even if you haven't had cancer, detoxification can be a wonderful tool for helping your body stay healthy. Detox is an integral part of living a cancer-prevention lifestyle. More and more we are able to link cancer to environmental exposures. And the best way to address these exposures is to remove as many as possible from your personal environment.

How are chemicals impacting your health?

One of the reasons cleansing is super important is because we all live in a pollution soup. I don't mean to be depressing, but it's true. Wherever you're sitting right now, even if it's a pristine environment out in the middle of the woods, you can probably point out some level of pollution. In wilderness areas, it's usually persistent solvents and pesticides that impact the "clean" water. In an average home, you could be exposed to cancer-promoting chemicals from the anti-dust spray you use to clean your coffee table, or from the pressboard furniture which has formaldehydes in it. Maybe you have scents in your home from candles or something that plugs into the wall, another common source of dangerous solvents and formaldehydes.

Super interesting when it comes to cancer is how toxins impair the immune system. I am always being asked: *What can I do to boost my immune system?* Fascinatingly, what tends to impair immune system function are the chemicals that are around us all the time.

Take, for instance, the research study that looked at Teflon. It showed the chemicals that come off of Teflon pans reduce natural killer cell response. Natural killer cells are essential for our immune system to respond to and get rid of cancer cells. Kind of important to know, right?

Chemicals can also disrupt hormone receptors. Certain

chemicals like bisphenol-A have been shown to stimulate estrogen receptors, potentially contributing to diseases like breast cancer, and reduce how effective treatments are for breast and prostate cancer.

Lastly, we have seen that heavy metals can also reduce natural killer cells.

Then there is electromagnetic pollution, which is an ever-present part of the pollution soup that we all live in. Electromagnetic pollution can include airplanes, x-rays, the sun and nuclear power plants. We also face low-frequency pollution, which includes cell phones, microwaves and electric blankets. You've probably heard about the importance of a digital detox and here you can see the extent of this kind of pollution in our lives.

There is currently an emerging discipline of study called environmental oncology that is gathering more information on how our day-to-day interactions with carcinogens are impacting our cancer risk, cancer growth, and even making cancer treatments less effective.

When do we start accumulating toxins?

Recent research has shown us that we start accumulating toxins in utero. When the egg and the sperm come together and create a zygote, which then becomes a fetus, we start accumulating toxins. Studies have even shown that the placenta, sperm, egg, and umbilical cord have toxins stored in them.

Other research studies have suggested that toxins don't affect you through just a single generation. At this time, toxins are thought to be traced back at least four generations. That means I'm not just my toxins, but I could also be carrying my mother's toxins, my grandmother's toxins, and my great-grandmother's toxins. This is why we can find things like DDT and flame retardants in blood samples of people who are not old enough to have been exposed to these chemicals.

Further to this, the genetic changes that happen from these toxins and toxic exposures are passed on for at least four generations.

The multi-generational effect of chemicals being passed on helps make up your *total body burden* of toxins. Total body burden sums up the amount of chemicals stored in your body from everything you have come in contact with. From bisphenol-A to phthalates, endocrine disruptors to heavy metals. Your tissue concentration of these chemicals increases over time. So as you build up these toxins in your system, your total body burden becomes heavier and heavier.

Your body is super smart and doesn't want all these toxins floating around in your system, so you store them. You have long-term and short-term storage of toxins that make up your body burden. Your long-term storage of your chemical body burden is found in your bones, fat, and blood. Your bones are responsible for storing heaving metals; fat cells for storing plastics and some pesticides; your blood for storing carbon monoxide. Your short-term storage of toxins is in urine.

With all that being thrown at us — and starting before we are even born! — cleansing seems like a no-brainer. But what's actually going on in our bodies when we detox?

What happens when we detox?

Let's start at the very beginning. The word "detoxification" is thrown around frequently in the media, in advertisements, and just about everywhere. Everyone is talking about detoxification, but what is it exactly?

Well, most simply put, detoxification is anytime that you're removing toxins from the body. That's kind of an obvious definition, but you probably want to know more, right? That's why we are going to dive deep into a little biochemistry right now, so stick with me here. On a deeper level what's happening with detoxification is that you are transforming toxic substances into less toxic substances. After this transformation, the toxins are removed through urine and bowel movements.

The problem with detoxification is that it can be easy to overload the liver during the process, and this causes a build-up of toxic substances or *metabolites*. If you've ever tried a detox or cleanse on your own and haven't felt that great, maybe you got headaches or brain fog, or just didn't feel like your best self, it's probably because you got the Phase 1 and Phase 2 detoxification system overloaded. You see, detoxing is a process, which we can separate into two phases and needs to be tackled in the right way. When overload happens, it can cause all kinds of negative side effects, which is why it's so important to learn how to detoxify in a way that best *supports* your body, and not just the way that it says to do it in a magazine, book, or back of a box in the health food store.

The liver is more complex than that back-of-a-packet approach. There are several different detoxification pathways that are important for transforming toxins.

The liver starts processing toxins using Phase 1 detoxification. Phase 1 detoxification is the first step to helping toxic chemicals and hormones get through the liver. Phase 1 detoxification is called the *enzymatic* phase and it includes the CYP450 system. The CYP450 system might sound like a lot of mumbo-jumbo to you, but I promise you have heard of it before… just not in the biochemical terms. The CYP system is what breaks down or metabolizes medications. When you've been told in the past to stay away from grapefruit when you take certain medications, it is because grapefruit could change the Phase 1 detoxification pathway and the CYP system.

In order for Phase 1 detoxification to work, it needs oxidation and reduction. When you hear the term *antioxidants*, it's usually because they support the first phase of detoxification.

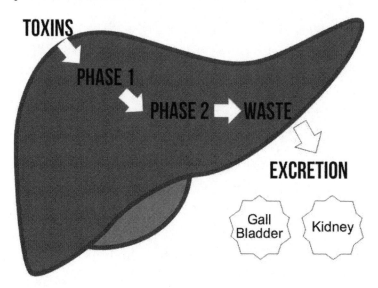

After Phase 1 detoxification, what you have are fat-soluble toxins. These fat-soluble toxins can get in kind of in a traffic jam between Phase 1 and Phase 2 detoxification if you have too many toxins being metabolized at once. This will cause the fat-soluble toxins to exit the liver and circulate to the rest of the body. One of the complications with a build-up between Phase 1 and Phase 2 is that hormone imbalance often happens here. It's also where carcinogens exit the liver and start circulating in the body.

Your body is pretty smart! It doesn't want all these toxins floating around, so you'll store them in your fat cells, in your muscle tissue, and in your brain. Yikes! That's why we want to ensure the Phase 1 to Phase 2 process goes smoothly. No traffic jams!

Next, we enter Phase 2 detoxification, which is called *conjugation*. This is what causes fat-soluble metabolites created in Phase 1 to become water-soluble. Once they are water-soluble, the toxins can be moved on as a waste product. These water-soluble waste products are excreted through the kidney and gallbladder.

Now, some people have a hard time with bowel movements and get constipation. If you are constipated or have experienced constipation in the past, this can cause a different kind of toxic traffic jam. When all is in good working order, the water-soluble waste products exit through bile from the gallbladder. However, if you have constipation, the liver detoxification pathway gets backed up. One of the benefits of having daily bowel movements is keeping this excretion pathway nice and open. One way bowel movements can be improved is by eating plenty of fiber. Fiber has the added benefit of absorbing certain toxins.

The other part of the Phase 2 detoxification to get these toxins completely out of your body is to ensure they exit through the kidneys and into your urine. When these toxic metabolites wind up in your urine, it is incredibly important for you to empty your bladder as often as you need to go. The longer the urine sits in the bladder with these toxic metabolites, the more time it has to come into direct contact with the bladder wall, which can make it more likely to damage the bladder wall and create problems.

Removing toxins through the urine is one of the reasons drinking plenty of water is so important during detox. You want to make sure that you can urinate and improve this excretion process. If you're dehydrated and only urinating once or twice a day, you might be backing up the excretion process through the kidneys.

The take-home message here is that you want to make sure you're urinating and having bowel movements regularly.

Supporting gentle detox

Some nutrients that are needed for Phase 1 detoxification include:

- B-vitamins

- Folic acid

- Glutathione

- Antioxidants

- Milk thistle

- Carotenoids

- Vitamin E

- Vitamin C

- Iron

- Magnesium

- Citrus bioflavonoids

- Quercetin

In Phase 2 detoxification, we're using nutrients like:

- Amino acids

- Glutathione

- Glycine

- Taurine

- Cysteine

- Sulfurated phytochemicals from garlic and cruciferous vegetables

Now that you understand the importance of detoxification, you can clean out some toxic storage in your body, just like you clean out your closet or garage. You have to move out the junk just to prevent your total body burden from getting overloaded and making you feel sick. Or worse yet, influencing your health to cause illness.

Detox? Cleanse? What's the difference?

So far I've been talking about both detoxing and

cleansing in this chapter. In fact, you may have heard *detoxing* and *cleansing* being used interchangeably out there in the world and be wondering what the difference is between the two.

Technically speaking, detoxification is the process of what's happening in the liver, as I just described above. Cleansing, also sometimes called *depuration*, is anytime we're freeing the body from something unwelcome. When we're doing a cleanse, we're using several different organ systems including the skin, the kidneys, the colon, the lungs, the lymphatic system, and the gallbladder.

Hopefully, all this biochemistry talk has helped you understand the importance of starting with a gentle cleanse. Almost everyone initially experiences a traffic jam between Phase 1 and Phase 2 detoxification, especially those who have gone through the oxidative stress of chemotherapy, surgery, and radiation. Even if you haven't had treatments for cancer, just living in this polluted world, you may see yourself going through the effects of a Phase 1 to Phase 2 detoxification traffic jam. We want to just gently support the toxin removal through the body to complete excretion.

How often should you cleanse?

I recommend cleansing a couple of times per year. If you want to be a cleansing rockstar, you can do a detox every quarter or season. The key, as I've mentioned, is gentleness and support.

Keep in mind that the way you support your body through a cleanse can be different depending on the season. For example, it feels way better to do a juice cleanse in the summertime when it's naturally hotter outside. Just like juicing feels better in the summer, warm foods can feel better in the winter. A winter cleanse could be a great time to focus on teas, soups and comforting vegan foods, for instance.

With all this background info, let's get started removing those impurities from your environment, home, and cells!

Cleansing your home

One of the first steps, but often overlooked parts of detoxification is removing toxic exposures from your day-to-day life. In naturopathic medicine, one of our primary principles is "prevention is the best cure." This means that your first step towards detoxification is to not get toxic exposures in the first place. Or to flip this on its head, what's the point of detoxing if you keep getting exposed to more toxins?

Going room by room is a simple way to clean up your environment. Your very first step is to make sure your chemical exposures become fewer and fewer. You are going to learn the most common chemical exposures one by one, room by room, so you can understand how to reduce them in your house and life overall. Picking just one room to start with can make the process so much easier.

Bathroom

Let's begin in the bathroom and talk about what's lurking in there. It's a lot more than stinky towels or mold! Your bathroom is where you get exposed to chemicals typically found in the soap aisle. Any typical grocery store smells like a fantastic floral arrangement chemical-style, but this chemical flower bouquet is the most common source of indoor air pollution and is what makes our indoor air pollution so much worse than outdoor air pollution.

Some of the substances that are in household cleaners and air scents include:

- Glycol ethers

- Alkylphenol ethoxylates

- Phthalates

- Triclosan

All of these items have been shown to cause nerve damage, infertility, disrupt hormone function, and form possible carcinogens.

In addition to the chemicals used to clean the bathroom, there are chemicals lurking in your skin care products, personal care products and soaps. Did you know that the average woman uses 12 personal care products daily? And the average man uses 6 products? On top of that, according to the Environmental Working Group, there are cancer-causing chemicals in one out of every five beauty products. These are shocking numbers! Apparently, it means the average woman is exposed to at least two cancer-causing chemicals every day! Can we agree that we can do better?

Common exposures from beauty and personal care products include:

- Heavy metals: sometimes used to color products like lipsticks, especially lead used for making red tones.

- Phthalates: this hormone-disrupting chemical is typically used to make fragrances and soaps.

- Xylene and toluene: what's jet fuel doing in your bathroom? These dangerous solvents are found in cosmetics like nail polish and nail polish removers.

- Sodium lauryl sulfate: this common surfactant (or soap latherer) has been linked to several types of cancer. In my house, this is a strict *avoid* chemical. It's hiding in your shampoo, body wash, and hand wash.

- 1,4–dioxane: this likely carcinogen is found in shampoo and cosmetics.

- Coal tar: this anti-dandruff ingredient could be considered a carcinogen.

- Triclosan: one of the most common disinfectants and anti-bacterial cleaners, and a possible carcinogen.

Bathroom solutions

At home, I'm always looking for alternatives. Here are some solutions that I use in my house, which I think you'll find super helpful to kickstart your home cleanse.

Dirt and soil dissolvers

If you're looking for something that can dissolve soil, this is going to sound way too simple, but I swear it's true! Try very hot water.

One of my favorite house-cleaning tips to share is simply putting on the tea kettle and keeping some piping hot water around. If there are any marks on the tiles or countertop, or anywhere that I'm cleaning, I can use this hot water to help dissolve any tough soil spots.

Looking for cleaners to help penetrate grime? There are some green alternatives that are based on soy or corn. If you're allergic to soy or corn, you can use coconut-based surfactants.

Antibacterial soap

Did you know that the most antibactieral substance is

just warm water and rubbing your hands together? In research studies looking at the benefits of soaps versus warm water and hand rubbing, they found the soap added little antibacterial efficacy. That means your best alternative to potentially toxic antibacterial soaps are warm water and friction. If you want to add a little extra oomph to this, try a soap that contains tea tree. This particular essential oil can be a great topical antibacterial agent.

Beauty products

One of the all-time greatest resources I've found for finding safe cosmetics or checking your cosmetics is *safecosmetics.org*. There are also apps for your phone like Dirty Girl, which can help you make decisions about products right when you are shopping. The Dirty Girl app lets you scan barcodes of the products you own or are about to buy, and tells you the chemicals they contain, their risks and benefits.

A simple swap with personal care products is to buy those that are fragrance-free. Even in a regular grocery store, Target, Wal-Mart, wherever you do your shopping, it's easy to find fragrance-free items.

I recommend using a nail polish that is formaldehyde-, toluene-, and xylene-free. Did you know that you can get this kind of nail polish at a normal beauty parlor? OPI is one of the brands that has pledged to be formaldehyde-, toluene-, and xylene-free and it is super easy to find, even at your local pedicure salon or beauty store.

Another great place to check your products is on the Skin Deep Cosmetics Database. If you have a smartphone, you can download the EWG Healthy Living app.

Living room

Let's talk about indoor air quality. Can you believe that indoor air has more pollutants in parts per million than our outdoor air? Incredible isn't it? And that doesn't matter where you're living, whether you are in New York or California or Colorado or Montana. Your indoor air has more pollution in parts per million than outdoor air.

Common indoor air pollutants include:

- Natural gas

- Oil

- Pressed wood

- Household cleaners

- Radon

- Pesticides

Air and dust samples contain:

- Plasticizers

- Disinfectants

- Flame retardants

- Persistent organic chloride pesticides

- Permethrin-based pesticides

The health effects of poor indoor air quality can include:

- Asthma

- Headaches

- Respiratory disease

- Heart disease

- Cancer

Living room solutions

Indoor air quality

No matter where you live, you want to make sure you dust and vacuum frequently, at least once a week if not more.

A study done on the east coast of the United States looked at what was contained in dust. When people dusted, they found that the particles of dust consisted of pesticides, herbicides, and heavy metals, so you want to make sure you're removing the dust on a regular basis.

Air quality also improves when you reduce solvents and chemical exposures in your home, by using cleaners that are more natural and less toxic, which we covered in the bathroom section.

One surprising yet interesting strategy that you can use to improve indoor air quality is to ventilate. No matter what time of year it is, no matter how cold or hot it is outside, your best move to improve air quality is opening your windows for at least 10 minutes every single day. This helps remove any air that's stagnant and toxic from inside your house, ventilating it to the outside and bringing in fresh air.

Windows seal incredibly well these days. (If you've updated your windows anytime recently, you'll know that you don't have to use your air conditioner or heater as much because you don't have as much air seeping in or out.) Because our homes have been so well sealed-off, the air is not moving at all inside. It stagnates. So fling open your windows and doors, and ventilate, ventilate, ventilate your home!

Another way you can improve indoor air is by using an air filter. An air filter can help reduce the parts per million of dusts, pesticides, solvents and chemicals. Look into which air filter is best for you.

Make sure, too, when you're buying any new furniture or bringing home dry cleaning, that you let it off gas outside before you bring it into your home. Here's how to do that. Hang the item in your backyard, garage, or someplace other than inside your closet or living room, wherever you're placing your new clothes or new furniture.

And finally, I believe what the astronauts don't know about air quality isn't worth knowing, which is why I look to them for inspiration! NASA has performed several studies examining the effective removal of volatile organic compounds (VOCs) from the air. The plants listed below are used in space stations to create safe breathing environments. You can apply this information at home to help improve your indoor air quality. Pretty cool, right?

- Bamboo palm

- Rubber plant

- Spider plant

- English ivy

- Schefflera

- Janet Craig Dracaena

- Dwarf date

- Boston fern

- Peace lily

Carpet freshener

Synthetic fragrances are one of the most concerning issues to me, and that's because they are a major hormone disruptor, which have been show to damage fish in the streams system. If synthetic fragrances are so damaging fish, just imagine what they're doing to us when we get *daily* toxic exposures.

Some green alternatives to synthetic fragrances include baking sodas and essential oil. I love sprinkling some baking soda on my carpets, with handfuls of dried lavender flowers, then vacuuming it all up. It just smells so lovely.

Kitchen

Let's shift focus to the kitchen. I've already mentioned some toxic exposures in the kitchen, such as Teflon pans, but let's look at a couple of other ways to make our kitchens a little less of a toxic hazard.

One of the main toxins that comes in through our kitchen is pesticide. Pesticides are neurotoxic and can add to the overall body burden of toxic chemicals. Pesticides are persistent in our environment, can cross the placental barrier, and are dangerous to preschoolers at high levels.

Browsing Facebook, I saw an awesome short film that looked into the pesticides in the urine of an entire family — mom, dad, brother, sister. The documentary examined their pesticide levels before and after going organic.

Before the experiment started, the family didn't eat anything organic. From the beginning of the experiment, they ate organic food only. The family's level of pesticides at the start was astonishing. Yet after they had gone organic, there were almost no detectable traces of pesticide in their urine.

Another published research study looked at the pesticide levels in the urine of preschoolers. In the urine samples, they were shown to have dangerously high levels of pesticides. It is thought that this comes down to high consumption of apples by preschooler's in apple slices, apple juice, and apple sauce. When the preschoolers had a single diet change of adding organic apples to their diet, the urine pesticide levels came down dramatically and they were no longer in danger zones of pesticide excretion.

That goes to show that simple and small changes can have an immediate effect. It's okay if you haven't been eating organic prior to reading this. Making a change now can have an instant impact.

Kitchen Solutions

Avoid pesticides

The "Dirty Dozen" is a list of fruits and vegetables to avoid, based on your likely pesticide exposure consuming them, which has been put together by the Environmental Working Group, an organization that looks at our environment and how it influences our health. I recommend you check out their website (www.ewg.org) if you haven't been on it before, because it's a great organization with informative resources particularly on this topic.

The Dirty Dozen changes every year or so, because the EWG is always re-testing to see what has the highest level of pesticides. To come up with the Dirty Dozen list, the EWG prepares the fruit or vegetables in the way that you would normally eat them. For instance, for bananas, they peel the banana, mash it up , and then measure the parts per million of pesticides in that banana. If they're testing an apple, on the other hand, they don't peel the apple because most of us eat the apple with the peel on. Then the apple gets mashed up and tested for parts per million of pesticides.

At the time of writing, the current Dirty Dozen is:

- Peaches

- Apples

- Sweet bell peppers

- Celery

- Nectarines

- Strawberries

- Cherries

- Lettuce

- Grapes (specifically imported)

- Pears

- Spinach

- Potatoes

They also put together a list called the Clean Fifteen, which right now are:

- Onions

- Avocados

- Sweet corn

- Pineapples

- Mango

- Papaya

- Honeydew melon

- Cantaloupe melon

- Sweet peas, frozen

- Asparagus

- Kiwi

- Cauliflower

- Cabbage

- Grapefruit

- Eggplant

This can be used to help prioritize what to buy organic and what you can buy conventionally grown. If something is part of the Cleanest Fifteen, then it's probably safer to buy non-organic than something that's on the Dirty Dozen list.

As indicated by the preschooler study, apples are a particular area of focus when we have young children or grandchildren. Make sure you're switching conventionally grown apples to organic apples to reduce the pesticide exposure level.

Taking off outdoor clothing

There are other ways to avoid pesticide exposure. One way to reduce the amount of pesticides that are trapped in the home and therefore your (and your pets') exposure to them is taking of your shoes as you enter your home. If you like wearing shoes inside of your home, keep one pair shoes for outside and a pair of slippers, flip-flops, or tennis shoes to wear indoors.

Remove clothing immediately after returning from parks, schools, farms and other sites of pesticide application. Parks and golf courses are common sources of pesticide exposure, especially when you're walking through the grass. Make sure you're taking off your clothing immediately after returning from golfing, if you enjoy golfing as a hobby.

Filtering it out

Try to avoid applying pesticides or herbicides in or around your home. Also make sure you're drinking filtered water because pesticides come through our water supply too.

Fruit and vegetable wash

Wash your non-organic produce in a hydrogen peroxide and water mix. Make sure you don't use too much hydrogen peroxide, because that can burn the throat and mouth. Just a little hydrogen peroxide can help remove any waxes or pesticides that are on the outside portion of your fruits and vegetables.

Change your cookware

Using glass, stainless steel, and cast iron can reduce exposure to Teflon and plastics.

Reduce heavy metal exposure

You can also use iodized salt to support thyroid function, eat low-mercury fish, and again make sure you filter your water. By changing your cookware to stainless steel and glass, you are also reducing your exposure to heavy metals like aluminum.

Digital detox

I know, I know. Going without our electronics feels
barbaric! I mean, it's one of the main sources of pleasure
in this day and age. But let's take a look at the science
from a health standpoint.

Our brains were designed to hold a certain amount of
information and decisions. However, according to
Alberto Villoldo, Ph.D, "From television and Internet
alone, we're exposed to more stimuli in a week than our
Paleolithic ancestors were exposed to in a lifetime." We
are now asking our brains to do in a week what it once
did in a *lifetime*. Pair that with the idea of how this
information we take in digitally impacts us. It's a lot to
think about!

As Kelly McGonigal, Ph.D. states, "Stress caused by the
news, as opposed to stress caused by your life, is unique
in its ability to trigger a sense of hopelessness... In fact,
a 2014 study of U.S. adults found that the single best
predictor of people's fear and anxiety was how much
time they spent watching TV talk shows." Maybe you
can relate to this. I know I can. My mom used to be
addicted to the news! She would get so upset by what
was happening in the world. Then as a way of processing
the grief, anger, and emotions elicited, she would call me
and tell me what was happening in the world. It got to a
place of getting teary and calling me every time a
tragedy, such as a global natural disaster, happened.

Maybe you have a family member like that. Someone who feels the world news so deeply that it causes an emotional reaction. Or maybe you are that relative. While it's beneficial to care about human wellness and actively support health and healing throughout the globe, you are creating an undue amount of stress by fixating on the news.

Did you know that people who watched 6+ hours of TV news about the Boston Marathon bombing experienced more post-traumatic stress than the people at the bombing?

As we say in my family, "News informs. It does not transform." This phrase helped my mom shake the news for good. Does she still stay informed about what's happening in the world? Absolutely. But she sees the need to participate actively in transformation through volunteer work, donations, and meditation. I'm proud of her for making this shift. And I know you can do it too!

Why is it so hard to let go of the news that *informs* us? Well, our brains are hard-wired to seek out new information. When we get a new piece of knowledge, our brain rewards us with dopamine, a feel-good brain chemical (and the same one released with cocaine use). To say that you might be addicted to information is not that far of a stretch.

When you take time out from your sources of information — the TV, your smartphone, the internet, social media — you are giving your brain time to sort and organize the other information that came to you that day, such as a smile from a loved one, a conversation with a stranger, the interaction with another driver while on the freeway.

Taking an informational or digital detox also provides the space to notice the little things, like the way the sunset looks tonight, how the breeze smells, and all the teeny tiny enjoyable parts of our environment that get drowned out by the daily digital noise. Allowing your brain more time and space to process and organize can allow you to become more focused and clear on what you truly want. What truly supports your best health? Your best mental function? Your best relationships?

When we use electronics, we can become easily distracted. Pulling away from the current moment or interaction by answering a text message, checking how many likes we got on our Facebook status, or digitally snooping on someone else. When we are distracted, we lose out on the opportunity for connected relationships, seeing the small beauty in everyday life, and hearing the whisperings of our higher soul.

How many times have I been in the car with a loved one, and instead of engaging in a conversation, I'm looking down at my phone writing a social media post? And if distraction takes us out of the present moment, digital technology can also help us avoid alone and quiet time.

Research studies have shown that when a mobile device is present, even if not in use, during a 10-minute conversation people reported lower levels of empathy and less friendliness towards each other. These people were not using their mobile devices; their phones were just sitting on the table! When a mobile device was not present during a 10-minute conversation, people were able to empathize with each other more. This is good backing for the "no phones at the table" rule. If you want your social interactions to be meaningful, put your mobile device away completely.

When you let go of extra information and distraction, a digital detox allows you to answer some important questions...

How are media posts and pictures influencing me to feel?

How do I react?

What is distracting me?

Let's do an exercise together. It might be a little uncomfortable, but it's an important part of cleansing. We are going to go through a couple of different digital technologies. When you look at each of these digital distractions, ask yourself:

- What draws me to this?

- What would I lose by giving it up?

- How can I replace this with some other type of behavior?

Then for each specific technology, ask these further questions:

Phone

- When do I reach for the phone? What's going on?

- What does the phone give me that I can't find within myself?

- How do I feel when I get off the phone?

TV

- What am I feeling while watching this show? Stress? Anger? Peace? Joy?

- Am I choosing programming consciously?

- What information does my DVR schedule reflect back to me?

- Has TV become a companion? A friend?

Apps and social media

- What am I feeling before I open it?

- What am I feeling while on this app?

Radio

- What am I thinking about when I reach for the radio power button?

- What emotion is the radio bringing into my environment?

- Am I avoiding anything when I listen to the radio?

Another side to the digital detox: EMF and EMR

After that last section, you are probably pretty clear on the emotional effects of the digital age. But what do you know about the cellular effects of the digital age? This is a whole different reason to avoid being all digital all the time!

One negative health influence of digital media is electromagnetic frequency (EMF) and electromagnetic radiation (EMR). Simply put, an electromagnetic field is generated when energy goes into motion. When a current flows from the power line to your house and out your electric socket, an electromagnetic field is being generated.

Why are people so concerned about EMFs and EMRs? Well, our exposure to electromagnetic fields and electromagnetic radiation has dramatically increased in the past couple of decades. Think about the number of electronic devices you use on a daily basis! From cell phones to alarm clocks, we are surrounded by electronics 24/7.

Is there a reason to be concerned? Probably. On the one hand, research studies show that low frequency electronic waves don't seem to impact somebody's health when exposed over a short period of time. But, we don't know what long-term exposure to low frequency waves will do. There is already some evidence that suggests it could be increasing childhood cancer rates. And the debate continues about cell phones and brain cancer.

What we do know about EMF and EMR exposure is that it can cause small currents of electricity to circulate in the body. We also know that radiofrequency and magnetic fields create a heating effect on body tissue. The main concern right now are power lines, cell phones, and cell phone signal towers. While the research is inconclusive, I recommend caution.

Here are five things you can do to reduce EMF and EMR exposure:

- **Use a headset.** Using a headset with your cell phone keeps the radiation further from your body.

- **Keep your phone out of the bedroom.** Cell phones emit more radiation when they are seeking out a signal versus when they are in use.

That means, when it's sitting on your nightstand, it has a higher level of radiation than when it is in use.

- **Plug in**. Wireless technology is one of main sources of daily EMR exposure. Cutting down on the wireless activity and using wired terminals is best for reducing exposures.

- **Practice grounding or earthing.** Grounding or earthing are practices that might seem a little new agey, but in all actuality, it has been suggested as a therapy for centuries! Earthing is the practice of bringing the frequency of your body to the same frequency of the earth. The easiest way to do this? Walking barefoot on wet grass or wet sand. This could be the reason why taking a walk on the beach can be so therapeutic.

- **Use shields.** There are many products for shielding against radiation and magnetic exposure. From window coverings, cell phone covers, to grounding cords for outlets, there are so many to choose from. I don't have favorite products right now, but as soon as I do, I'll be sure to let you know!

If you are on my e-mail list, you will hear about every discovery I make in this area and how to protect yourself. You can sign up for more EMF information at: http://drheatherpaulson.com/bookresources/

Light pollution

Did you know that 63% of the global population and 99% of population of the United States and European Union experience light pollution? Have you ever wondered what the outdoor street lamps emitting light at night are doing to your health? If not, it's time to start!

Here are a couple of ways that artificial light at night has been shown to change health:

- Disrupting your day/night cycle (also known as *circadian rhythm*)

- Changing your brain chemistry and function

- Increasing tumor growth

- Causing sleep disorders

- Changing melatonin production

While the link between light and sleepless nights might be an easy leap to make, what about too much light being linked to cancer growth? Not so intuitive! Research studies have identified that night shift workers are at higher risk of breast cancer and colon cancer. But what does that mean for ambient light from living in a city? Honestly, we don't know yet. But it's pretty easy to reduce your light exposure at nighttime... So why not do it until research is more conclusive? I'll give you a few suggestions of how to cleanse this area of your life shortly.

Another piece of the light puzzle is melatonin. This hormone is suppressed when you are exposed to light. Melatonin is important in helping your immune system function, particularly the part of your immune system that is responsible for tagging and getting rid of cancer cells. We want this hormone to be working properly!

There are other genes regulated by the day/night cycle too. These genes are called *clock genes* and are responsible for making proteins that impact your overall health, not just cancer risk. Light pollution has also been linked to:

- Weight gain

- Depression

- Anxiety

- Diabetes, especially in women

- Headaches

- Weakened vision

- High blood pressure

Here are 10 ways you can reduce light pollution impact on your health:

- Avoid shift work.

- Sleep in a room that has blackout curtains.

- Cover the light emitted from alarm clocks and other light-emitting items in your bedroom.

- Switch outdoor lights to be motion-sensor only.

- Use light fixtures approved by International Dark Sky Association.

- Download an app for your computer and phone that makes the display screen mimic outdoor light rhythms; try f.lux, Lux, and Twilight.

- Avoid blue light. This light wave has been associated with poorer health in particular. When looking for new light bulbs, choose ones that have a warmer hue and are less white in color, specifically a color temperature of 3500K or lower.

- Use dimmer switches on indoor lights. This allows you to reduce the amount of light exposure you have after dusk and before dawn.

- Talk to your power company and city about dark sky initiatives.

- Turn off the lights. By limiting light exposure, you are limiting light pollution. You can also opt for softer light from lamps.

Start cleansing!

Now that we have covered all your exposures in day-to-day life and how to reduce your exposure, we can move into how to gently mobilize toxins stored in your system. Getting started with a cleanse can be intimidating and potentially depleting. That's why I suggest that you start gently, and with the approval of your doctor. A gentle cleanse is a way to slowly introduce cleansing practices into your everyday life. Gentle cleansing can allow you to build up your vitality, reduce negative reactions that you might have, or gradually eliminate certain chemicals in your environment. In my opinion, this is the best way to start detoxing after cancer treatment.

The best way to start a gentle cleanse is by increasing water intake. This is the very first change you can apply and it's easy. By improving hydration, you are shifting how toxins move out of your body through the kidneys. If you don't like the taste of water, you can always add mint, ginger, or lemon to it. As a bonus, these herbs, roots, and citrus can help your body with the detoxification process.

Don't forget, you can also use herbal teas as an opportunity to support liver and kidney function in a gentle cleanse. Some teas I recommend to my patients are dandelion and burdock root. Dandelion can be a great coffee substitute, because it has a similar bitterness flavor profile to coffee, while also helping you let go of caffeine.

Another way to start gentle cleansing is to use more liver supportive foods in your diet daily. These foods include cruciferous vegetables, sprouts, beets, whole grains, and leafy greens. You can add in kidney support such as cranberries, beans, and magnesium-rich foods too.

Supporting the lymphatic system is critical when talking about gentle cleansing. The lymphatic system supports the immune system, filters waste, and transports fluid from our intracellular spaces to circulation. Unlike arteries, the lymphatic system doesn't have a pump. So it relies on movement of the muscles to create movement in lymphatic fluid. In gentle cleansing, the lymphatics can be stimulated with dry skin brushing, gentle exercise, and even rocking in a rocking chair.

One of the body's largest organs of detoxification is often underestimated and overlooked. It's the skin. The skin assists the removal of toxins via sweat. One way I encourage patients to use sweating in detoxification is through a sauna. Studies looking at the contents of sweat droplets following an infrared sauna session have shown to contain pesticides, herbicides, heavy metals, and solvents. Sauna is a great way to mobilize the toxins that are stored in our fat cells in particular and get rid of them via the skin.

Our skin can absorb toxins too, though, so think about what you are placing on your skin and absorbing throughout the day. Go back to the list of bathroom-based toxins and check your products are free of these chemicals.

In a gentle cleanse, you can support elimination through the colon as well. It is recommended to have a daily bowel movement, but not through means that are forceful. Every day you don't have a bowel movement, you're reabsorbing toxins. Some gentle ways to encourage bowel movements is through introducing more fiber into your diet, especially in the form of flaxseeds, chia seeds, psyllium, and chicory. If chronic constipation has been a health issue for you, do talk to your healthcare team about this.

Castor oil packs applied topically are one gentle cleansing technique that can be used to support cleansing through the liver and the abdomen. The way that you use castor oil is strictly topical, because if you take it internally, it can potentially be toxic. Saturate a flannel cloth completely with the castor oil pack and then you apply that cloth over the liver or intestines. On top of that, place a heating pad, then rest and relax for 20-40 minutes. Ensure you don't apply heat in any areas of your body that may have neuropathy or difficulties sensing temperature.

In a gentle cleanse, it's important also to support the lungs. The lungs are important for deep breathing. Every time we exhale, we release a build-up of CO_2 and other toxins. There are ancient yoga practices that involve breathing and I highly recommend watching the bonus videos on how to use pranayama (breathwork) in your everyday life: http://drheatherpaulson.com/bookresources/

One of my favorite tools for implementing pranayama at home is an app by Saagara that you can download for your smartphone or simply use on your computer to guide you through the inhalation and exhalation process of breathing.

Cleanse overview

Before starting a cleanse, please talk to your doctor to see what is safe for you and your body. It's an important piece of care to individualize a cleanse strategy for you and your health goals.

Week 1: Getting prepped

It's all in the preparation! Choose your cleanse strategy and start reducing your caffeine intake by 50%. Eliminate fried foods. Start introducing honey, molasses, and maple syrup as sweeteners. Start to minimize red meat intake.

Week 2: Elimination phase

Eliminate all of the following foods:

Milk, cheese, eggs, all wheat products, citrus fruits, tomatoes, potatoes, corn and corn products, peanuts, peanut butter, coffee, all caffeinated teas, alcohol, red meat, pork, sugar, NutraSweet, and all sweeteners (except maple syrup and honey), fried foods, any processed food.

Start replacing one meal a day with a protein shake or adding a protein shake as a snack. Reduce fruit to two servings daily.

Week 3: Continue elimination, intensify cleansing practices (optional)

If choosing a more intense cleanse, start replacing two meals with a protein shakes. Add 1 or 2 days of juice and protein powder only based on what you committed to during Week 1. You can also completely eliminate all sweeteners. Reduce fruit to one serving daily.

Week 4: Adding back

Start adding back foods one category at a time every 72 hours. That means you can add in several dairy products in one day, and see how your body responds.

Week 5: Re-establish

Re-establish a diet that feels good for you.

Some ways to intensify the third week of cleansing are the I'm Too Tired to Cleanse cleanse, the Weekend Warrior cleanse, and the Clear Out The Junk cleanse.

The I'm Too Tired To Cleanse cleanse

The I'm Too Tired To Cleanse cleanse is the simplest and gentlest version of a cleanse. This kind of cleanse involves eliminating caffeine, alcohol, wheat, dairy, soy, sugar and corn. You don't even have to eliminate all of them; you can just eliminate one of them. You could also add in one cleansing activity to your routine every week for four weeks. This cleanse could also include removing one toxic exposure from your home every week for four weeks. Your goals while on the I'm Too Tired To Cleanse cleanse are:

- Drink water and stay hydrated.

- Try adding one new cleansing food every week for four weeks.

- Avoid new toxic exposures and pick one thing to remove from your home every week for four weeks.

- Add in one cleansing activity to your routine every week for four weeks.

- Eliminate at least one of the following foods: coffee, alcohol, wheat, dairy, soy, sugar, corn.

The Weekend Warrior cleanse

During Week 3 of a cleanse, you might choose to do a two- or three-day Weekend Warrior cleanse, where you eliminate all processed foods for at least three days. You drink plenty of water and stay hydrated and then you add in one or two cleansing activities to your routine whether that's a bath, dry skin brushing, or sauna. With the Weekend Warrior cleanse, you could also do a castor oil pack nightly.

You can extend the Weekend Warrior cleanse to be Seven-Day cleanse. We can get through just about anything for a week, although I'm not advocating for your suffering, even for five to seven days.

During this week, eliminate all processed foods, dairy, sugar, coffee, alcohol and soda. Take out meat completely and eat a vegan diet. After the week, you can add back processed foods, dairy, sugar, coffee, alcohol, and soda if you choose. During the cleanse, make sure to stay well hydrated and add in one or two cleansing activities to your routine every day.

Your goals during a Weekend Warrior cleanse are to:

- Eliminate all processed foods for three full days.

- Drink water and stay hydrated.

- Add in a couple cleansing activities to your routine every day.

- Drink one green juice every day.

Your goals during the Seven-Day cleanse are:

- Day 1 and 2: Eliminate all processed foods, dairy, sugar, coffee, alcohol, soda, and meat except fish.

- Day 3: Have a completely vegan diet.

- Day 4 - 5: Repeat Days 1 and 2.

- Drink water and stay hydrated.

- Drink green juice once or twice a day.

- Add in a couple cleansing activities to your routine every day.

The Clear Out The Junk cleanse

There's also the Clear Out The Junk cleanse, where you go all in. It is a 10-day cleanse where you eliminate all processed foods, dairy, sugar, coffee, alcohol, and soda. Eliminate meat for two days. Then add back in the processed foods, dairy, sugar, coffee, alcohol and soda after eliminating meat and eating a largely vegan diet for several days.

Your goals during the Clear Out The Junk cleanse are:

- Day 1 to 3: Eliminate all processed foods, dairy, sugar, coffee, alcohol, soda, and meat except fish.

- Day 4 to 6: Eat a wholly vegan diet.

- Day 7 to 10: Repeat Days 1 to 3.

- Drink water and stay hydrated.

- Drink green juice once or twice a day.

- Add in a couple cleansing activities to your routine every day.

During this first week of a cleanse, it's important to reduce overwhelm by focusing on a few key points. The first aspect to tackle is reducing caffeine. Start thinking about your current caffeine intake whether that's zero coffee or 12 cups of caffeine. Just check in with yourself and see where your caffeine intake is, then cut this down by at least 50% over the next seven days.

You might also focus on eliminating: fried foods, sugar and artificial sweeteners, all artificial colors and flavors. And reducing: red meat to once or twice a week, processed foods to less than or equal to 50% of your meal. While increasing: water intake to at least eight cups per day if it is safe for your kidneys, detoxification supplements that have been approved by your healthcare team.

The first week of a cleanse is a great time to start experimenting with new foods, spices, and oils in your diet. That way, once you start letting go of more foods in the coming weeks, you already have some delicious options for replacements.

Your cleanse checklist

If your doctor okays a cleanse, here are some of the items you'll want to gather before starting. It's great to have these on hand and ready to go! This will help you set yourself up for success.

Again, be sure to check with your doctor that cleansing is safe for you. As a naturopathic doctor, I respect that each individual is unique. Following a predetermined program without discussing it with someone who can guide you could lead to health problems. For my patients, I customize this program to meet their individual needs and current health goals.

Groceries

- Protein powder

- Digestive enzyme

- Greens powder

- Amino acid blend

- Water bottle

- Blender or blender bottle

- Whole grains (rice, buckwheat, bulgur, etc)

- Veggies that you can cut up for snacks

- Nuts or trail mix that is not sweetened

- Nut butter (almond, cashew)

- Low glycemic fruit: berries, cherries, prunes, dried apricots, apples, peaches

- Milk alternatives: cashew, almond, coconut

- Gluten-free crackers

- Decaf/herbal tea

- Canned or dried beans

- Fish such as salmon, mahi mahi, ono

- Coconut oil

- Olive oil

- Real maple syrup

- Curry powder or other favorite spice blends

Household/lifestyle items

- Salt scrub for bath/shower (see recipes under hydrotherapy section)

- Journal

- Essential oils, especially lavender, lemon

- Supportive friends

- Dry skin brush

- Favorite teacup

You can also enhance your cleanse with supplements. To learn more about the supplement packs my patients use, and for some extra cleanse recipes, visit the website here: http://drheatherpaulson.com/bookresources/

Keeping it tasty!

Here's what you can add to that shopping list to make sure you're keeping your cleanse tasty and appealing.

- Spices (also the best way to keep your food tasting lovely!)

- Oil: coconut oil, olive oil

- Sweeteners: honey, stevia, maple syrup

- Poultry: free range, organic only

- Fish: deep sea fish

- Legumes: lentils, split peas, pinto beans, kidney beans, soy beans, mung beans, adzuki beans

- Grains: millet, basmati, brown rice, quinoa, amaranth, oatmeal, barley, buckwheat, teff

- Steamed vegetables

- Herbal teas

- Water

Common side effects of cleansing

Anytime you change your diet, there might be a couple of symptoms that make your experience less than pleasant. These suggestions are to help get you through so you can feel all the health benefits of doing a cleanse!

Gas and bloating

- Chew, chew, chew! Now that you are eating more fiber and starches, your stomach depends on the enzymes in your mouth to break down the food.

- Soak and rinse beans (even canned beans).

- Spice it up! Use ginger, fennel seeds, and mint to reduce bloating.

- Take an enzyme supplement like the d-tox digest that's included in my detox supplement kit. You can learn more here: http://drheatherpaulson.com/bookresources/

Headaches

- Drink plenty of fluids.

- If it is a caffeine withdrawal, add in products that are lower in caffeine such as green tea or black tea.

- Eat frequently throughout the day. You may be experiencing blood sugar changes.

- Focus on magnesium-rich foods, like leafy greens and nuts. Consider adding a magnesium supplement.

- Focus on B-vitamin-rich foods, like whole grains, nutritional yeast. Consider adding a B-complex.

- Focus on tryptophan-rich foods: tofu, lentils,

nuts, seeds, black beans, kidney beans, brewer's yeast.

Fatigue

- Make sure you are eating enough!

- Focus on energy and amino-acid-rich foods: hemp, sprouts, and leafy greens.

- Eat foods that are an instant source of energy: bananas, berries, dates, mango, figs, pineapple, berries.

Irritability

- Focus on tryptophan-rich foods: tofu, lentils, nuts, seeds, black beans, kidney beans, brewer's yeast.

- Eat small frequent meals. Don't go hungry!

Changes in bowel movements

Constipation:

- Since you're adding more fiber to your diet, make sure you are matching this with an equal amount of fluids.

- Trying decreasing breads and processed grains. Increase foods rich in enzymes such as papaya, pineapple, and apple cider vinegar.

- Add chia or flax seeds which provide stool lubrication.

Diarrhea:

- Add in more processed grains and rice.

- Reduce raw foods or use vinegar to help break down raw foods prior to eating.

- Reduce meat substitutes and cheese substitutes. Stick to whole foods.

- Eat an apple daily; the fiber in apple helps bind the stool together.

Dairy and cheese cravings

- Recognize that dairy stimulates an opiate response... It's addictive!

- Try tahini dressings, hummus, and raw nut "cheeses": these foods taste like cheese and provide the nutrients needed to balance your brain chemistry as you withdraw from cheese.

- Try a nut-based milk (almond, hazelnut, etc).

Home practices

Often, I hear people say that they can't cleanse because they have bad reactions to the supplements or making the diet changes are just too hard. But guess what! There are simple little changes just about anybody can make throughout the day to help the body cleanse.

Introducing cleansing *practices* allows you to make cleansing a part of your daily health routine instead of limiting it to an annual or seasonal event. You certainly don't have to do all of these, but maybe just pick out one or two and incorporate it into your daily routine.

Hydrotherapy

Hydrotherapy is one of my all-time favorites, especially doing this at home. Personally, I try to do some type of hydrotherapy treatment at least once a week. It helps keep my body and immune system in tip top function. The simplest form of hydrotherapy, or using water to heal yourself naturally, is taking a bath or shower (and hopefully you are doing this more than once a week already!)

A word of caution… Hot water hydrotherapy is not recommended if you have any heart issues because it might alter blood pressure or heart rhythm. It should also be used cautiously with lymphedema. If you have any concerns, please check with your doctor.

Why do hot baths work? Hot water draws toxins out of the body to the skin's surface. As the water cools, it pulls the toxins from the skin. Epsom and other salts augment this detoxification by causing you to sweat, while also providing an alkaline and cleansing medium. Here are a few ingredients you can try adding to your bath to aid the toxin elimination and also make the hydrotherapy session oh-so pleasurable.

Epsom salt

Commonly used for sore muscles, this salt is high in magnesium and sulfur. Both of these nutrients are needed for both Phase 1 and Phase 2 detoxification in the liver. Your body absorbs the nutrients through the skin while you sit in the bathtub.

Baking soda

You might also want to use baking soda in your bath. Baking soda has been thought to be alkalinizing and may help alkalinize the body through the skin. It has traditionally been used to treat rashes and skin irritation.

Coffee

You have probably thought that coffee is only for drinking, but I'm here to bust that myth! Coffee is a great plant to use topically. One of the awesome benefits of coffee is that is can help reduce skin cancer when applied to the skin.

Usually, I will add a cup of coffee into my bath, especially when I'm being exposed to more sun than usual. It's a great bath to take after being on a hike, working in the garden, or having some time at the beach.

A word of caution with coffee: it can be over-stimulating! If you stay in a coffee bath for too long, you can absorb some of the caffeine through your skin.

To avoid staining your bath tub a coffee color, put some bubble bath in before adding the coffee. It made all the difference in my house when I figured out this trick! My husband wasn't left with a coffee ring around the bathtub, which made him happy.

Ginger

Another great way to enhance your bath is to add in herbs, an incredible one to try being ginger. Ginger is a diaphoretic, which means it makes your blood vessels open and can increase sweating. Adding ginger makes bath time a little spicy, and you might feel the warmth tingling on your skin. Don't be surprised if ginger makes you start to sweat it out! It's one of the benefits. Because of its warming and diaphoretic action, avoid this bath if you have any issues with your heart.

Clay

Bentonite clay has been shown to draw out impurities. It's easily found at the health food store for this exact purpose. To use clay, take about a quarter cup of the clay and mix it into your bathtub. Soak in your bath as usual. Full disclosure… This is messy!

Peat moss

Peat moss, which is typically used in your planters to make a nice mossy top for your plants, has been shown to bind to heavy metals and is a great addition for hydrotherapy. Now, you don't want to buy the peat moss from your local home warehouse store, of course! Make sure you're getting peat moss that's specifically for hydrotherapy with no added chemicals.

Seaweed

Okay, I know this sounds kind of crazy, but I love adding seaweed to my bath. I have no doubt you will too if you give it a try! Using seaweed that's in a package (like kombu), add 1 to 4 leaves to your bath tub as the water is filling. Full of essential minerals, seaweed is nourishing to the skin, while providing nutrients needed for detoxification.

Basic salt soak

Minerals and salts make the bath water feel silky, and leave your skin cleansed and soft.

1 cup of sea salts

2 cups of baking soda

1 cup of Epsom salts

1 to 2 tbsp of glycerin or Dr. Bronner's Soap per bath

Combine the sea salts, baking soda, and Epsom salts in a bowl. Stir to blend. Pour a quarter of a cup or so into the bath while the tub is filling. Add 1 to 2 tablespoons (more for dry skin, less for oily skin) of glycerin or Dr.

Bronner's Soap to keep your skin from drying out and essential oils of choice.

Preparation time: 2 to 3 minutes

Shelf life: indefinite

Storage: glass jar with a screw top

Caution: Do not take hot baths or salt baths (including Epsom salt baths) if you have heart trouble, high blood pressure, or are diabetic.

Essential oils

- **Geranium:** This is one of the best essential oils for the skin. It stimulates the liver and kidneys, aids the immune system and promotes blood circulation. Its soothing aroma makes it perfect to blend with angelica, grapefruit or orange.

- **Grapefruit:** Grapefruit helps with the regulation of fluids. It stimulates the lymphatic system and aids with water retention. Its refreshing scent makes it an ideal mood-lifter too. Just be careful about going in the sun afterwards, as it can make your skin photosensitive.

- **Lemon:** Like lemon juice, lemon essential oil can help your body to detox naturally. It is known to support the liver and kidneys as well as promoting blood circulation and strengthening the immune system.

- **Lavender:** A nervous system tonic, lavender is known for its ability to bring down stress hormones and soothe the soul. If stress is an emotion you are detoxing from, lavender will be a great companion.

Detox showers

Don't like taking baths or don't have a bathtub available? Don't worry! You can do a detox shower too. One of the easiest ways to use some of the bath ingredients in a shower is to make a salt scrub.

Coffee salt scrub

1½ cups of coarse sea salt

1 cup of freshly ground or pre-ground coffee

1 cup of oil of your choice (such as coconut, olive, apricot, avocado)

5 to 15 drops essential oil (optional)

In a large bowl, add coarse sea salt and coffee grounds. Stir together. Add oil and essential oil and stir. Store in an airtight container.

Caution: Can be slippery when used in a shower, so please be careful.

Lavender salt scrub

1 cup of table salt or coarse sea salt

1 cup of coconut oil (or another oil of your choice) or glycerin soap

20 drops lavender essential oil

Add salt, coconut oil, and essential oil to a large bowl. Mix together until well combined. Store in an airtight container.

Again, this can make the shower slippery, so take care.

Contrasting shower

A contrasting shower can improve circulation and vitality. It can also promote detoxification and elimination. This is a great way to finish your salt scrub after rinsing off completely. Here's how you do it:

Step 1: Stand in warm/hot water for 3 to 5 minutes.

Step 2: Stand in cold/cool water for 30 seconds to 1 minute. This can take courage! If cold water is too much, you can start by just using a temperature that's cooler than your version of warm.

Step 3: Repeat going from hot to cold two or three times. Always ending on cold.

Foot bath

Foot baths are another way to utilize hydrotherapy without a bath or a shower. Traditionally used to relieve headaches, congestion, swelling, and fatigue. You will need a couple of household items to do this, but it's pretty simple. If you have any peripheral neuropathy, this cleanse habit is not recommended for you.

2 buckets

2 towels

Total time: 10 to 15 minutes

In bucket 1, fill with warm/hot water to tolerance, leaving some room at the top. Take care to not burn yourself. In the second bucket, add cool/cold water. For the brave at heart, you can even add ice!

Step 1: Place buckets 1 and 2 on top of one of the towels on the floor.

Step 2: Put your feet in the warm bucket up to mid-calves for 3 to 5 minutes.

Step 3: Take feet out of the first bucket and move to the cold bucket for 30 seconds to 1 minute.

Step 4: Repeat Steps 1 and 2 twice more.

Step 5: Dry feet applying friction with the towel.

Lymphatic movement

During a cleanse, it's critical to support the lymph system. The lymphatics are responsible for immune function, filtering bacteria, and clearing out cellular debris. The lymphatic system is composed of lymph vessels, lymph nodes, and organs.

Our blood vessels use the heart as a pump to deliver blood throughout your body. The lymphatic system uses the movement of your skeletal muscles to pump lymph fluid throughout your body. No muscular movement equals no lymphatic movement!

Lucky for you, helping your lymphatic system can be simple. You don't need a fancy rebounder or trampoline (although I think that's a pretty fun option too!) Let's take a look at some of your options.

Rocking

Yes! Pumping the lymphatic system can be as simple as rocking in a rocking chair! One porch side swing coming right up! Rocking in a rocking chair for 10 to 15 minutes per day can help utilize your lower leg muscles to pump the lymph back up towards the heart.

Lymphatic massage

You can go to a special massage therapist for a lymphatic massage. This is a gentle massage with broad strokes. If you can't make it to the spa regularly, another option is to perform a self-lymphatic massage. For clear instructions, go to the cleanse website to watch the video showing you how to do this.

Dry skin brushing

Stimulating the lymphatic system through dry skin

brushing can activate lymph function as well as encourage blood circulation and cell regeneration. Skin brushing can also provide exfoliation, stimulate sebaceous glands for improved skin moisture, and improve sweating.

Supplies needed are just a natural bristle brush, preferably with a long handle. If you can't find a natural bristle brush, you can use a loofah or dry wash cloth.

Step 1: Start by gently brushing your feet, including the soles. Move upwards to the thighs in small circular motions. Keep moving upward until you hit the belly button.

Step 2: Brushing towards the heart, raise one arm up and brush towards the armpit. Repeat on the other arm.

Step 3: Brush over the breast, around neck, and shoulders.

Step 4: Brush abdomen from left to right and in a circle.

Exercise

During detoxification, it is best to rest or do light exercise and avoid overexertion. It does not take extreme stimulation to get the lymphatic system pumping. Some beneficial exercises that will help with elimination are:

- Light walking

- Light stretching

- Gentle yoga

- Light walking in a swimming pool

Please do not overdo exercising! We live in a society where pushing our bodies harder and doing exercise extremes like bootcamp, spin class, or crossfit is seen as desirable. Cleansing is about resting and rejuvenation. A little gentle movement goes a long way!

If you have a hard time resting or backing down your exercise routine, ask yourself: *What am I getting out of extreme exercise? What is it doing for me emotionally? Is this balanced or unbalanced?*

If you have a hard time getting started with exercise, ask yourself: *What are the messages keeping my body from moving? Is it pain, fear, resentment? What is not exercising doing for me emotionally? Is this balanced or unbalanced?*

Cleansing emotionally

It is common for emotions such as anger, sadness, and irritability to rise to the surface while cleansing. As you strip away from foods that soothe your emotions to nourishment and practices that heal, you might find that old thought patterns, emotions, and habits come to the surface. You might also notice an increased sensitivity to the outside world. This is a great time to relax into these patterns with quiet introspection, self-nourishment, and down time.

Some helpful practices to gain insight or promote relaxation can be: journaling, meditation, breathing exercises, body scans, counseling, art projects, essential oils.

Journaling

Journaling can be an important tool for reflection and review. It allows us to integrate our experiences from the day. You might love journaling, or you might think journaling is kind of hokey and best left to junior high girls. Whatever your belief, I invite you to try journaling during this cleanse experience and see how it serves or doesn't serve you.

For journaling prompts and pages specifically designed for cleansing at all levels go to http://drheatherpaulson.com/bookresources/. You can follow the prompts or journal whatever is on your mind.

Body scans

The guided meditation practice of body scanning allows you to see where certain emotions are impacting your physical health. You can become more attuned with areas of your body that have been walled off or injured.

The recorded guided meditation that comes with this cleanse is one example of a body scan. If you would like to practice a body scan without the recording, you can follow these simple steps.

Step 1: Take a seated or lying position, and close your eyes.

Step 2: Allow your body to settle into the ground if you are lying flat or into the chair if you are in a seated position. You might feel yourself grounded and connected to the earth through your feet, your tailbone, and your legs. As you connect to the earth the body begins to feel a little heavier.

Step 3: In your mind, flow from body part to body part, lingering for only 2 to 5 seconds at each place.

As you are prompted, move on to the next body part. Do not linger on one body part and do not worry if you can't feel any sensations in some areas of the body. We are just gathering information from our body without expectations or judgment.

Pass your awareness over your body starting from your head...

Feel your face. Notice your jaw, your mouth. Your left cheek, your right cheek. Your tongue. Your teeth. Your top teeth, your bottom teeth. All the parts of your mouth.

Feel your nose. Your right nostril, your left nostril. Feel the breath passing in and out of your nostrils. Feel the sensation of the breath through your nose, the temperature, the moisture. Feel your nose.

Moving to the sides of your head, feel your ears. Bring

awareness to the left ear, then the right ear. You notice the folds of the ear, the lobes, the ear canals. You are aware of your ears receiving sound. Feel your ears.

Feel your eyes, your eyelids, eyelashes, deep into the eye socket where your eyeball is cradled. Feel your eyes.

Move your awareness to your forehead, crown, whole head. Down to the throat, the neck.

Your right shoulder, right arm, right wrist, right hand, and right palm. Feel each finger starting with the thumb and moving to the pinky. Feel your right hand receiving energy through the palm from the surrounding air. Almost like you can feel a vibration or tingling of energy. Bring that energy back up the arm to the throat.

Move to the left shoulder. Feel the left shoulder, elbow, forearm, wrist, palm. Feel each finger starting with the thumb and moving to the pinky. Feel your right hand receiving energy through the palm from the surrounding air. Almost like you can feel a vibration or tingling of energy. Bring that energy back up the arm to the throat.

Bring that energy from the neck down to the chest. Feel your heart, the gentle beating of your heart. Feel the chest cavity, your lungs as they expand with the inhale and deflate with the exhale. Feel your shoulder blades, and ribs.

The awareness moves down from the chest to the belly button, the stomach, the intestines. Down to the lower back.

Notice the hips. The right hip, the right thigh, the right knee, right lower leg, right ankle, top of the foot, arch of the foot. Notice each toe starting at the big toe and moving to the smallest toe. Feel your whole right foot rooted and grounded into the earth through the sole.

Bring that energy from the sole of the foot back up to the belly button. Then become aware of your left hip. Move the awareness to the left thigh, knee, and lower leg. Left ankle, left top of the foot, left arch of the foot. Notice each toe starting at the big toe and moving to the smallest toe. Feel your whole left foot rooted and grounded into the earth through the sole.

Step 4: To finish the body scan, bring your awareness to the whole right side of your body. Then feel the left side. Feel the front of your body. And then feel the back of your body. Feel the whole body together. Feel the connection of all these parts that come together to make up the one and only you.

Step 5: Deepen your breath. Inhale. Exhale. See your whole body bathed in golden light. Each cell is given the space and energy to heal.

Step 6: Come back to the room. Come back to your body. Wiggle your fingers and toes. Open your eyes with a great big smile.

Art projects

Creativity is a great way to access emotions, hopes, fears, and dreams that might not otherwise bubble to the surface. Art allows you to reconcile emotional conflicts, increase self-awareness, reduce anxiety, and improve self-image.

When my husband and I were recovering from his cancer, one activity that helped us express our feelings about the whole experience was art therapy led by a counselor in a cancer support group. If there are emotions holding you back, but you're not sure how to express them, consider art therapy with a local facilitator.

There are so many ways to get started using art, from vision boards to coloring books! Pick an art form that resonates with you and just get started. Personally, I love mixed media. Getting my hands dirty with magazine clippings, glue, and glitter taps into that inner child where self-expression is done just for the fun of it!

Breathwork

One often-overlooked organ of detoxification is your lungs. Using the lungs during your cleanse allows you to exhale toxins, negative emotions, and anything else holding you back.

In yoga, the use of breathwork for healing is called *pranayama*. There are several detoxifying breaths to choose from, including: breath of fire, lion's breath, and nadi shodhana.

Now, it might seem kind of oversimplified to use breathing, something you do every minute of every day, to detoxify your system. However, these breathing exercises are potent and have been used to improve health for centuries. Deep breathing helps to calm and rejuvenate the nervous system, increase the mind's ability to focus, and restore balance in the different hemispheres of your brain.

We will cover two basic breathing sequences that are the safest breaths to use for most people. Anytime you start retaining your breath, it can cause dizziness or shortness of breath. If you begin experiencing these symptoms, stop the breathing exercise immediately and start breathing normally.

Nadi shodhana (alternate-nostril breathing)

Step 1: Take a comfortable seat. Make sure your spine is tall and straight, and your chest lifted and open.

Step 2: Bring your right pointer finger to the right nostril. Close your eyes and take a deep breath in your left nostril.

Step 3: Hold your breath for 3 seconds.

Step 4: Place your left index finger to the left nostril. Remove the right finger.

Step 5: Exhale out the right nostril.

Step 6: Hold for 3 seconds at the bottom.

Step 7: Inhale through the right nostril.

Step 8: Hold for 3 seconds.

Step 9: Place your right index finger to the right nostril. Remove the left finger.

Step 10: Exhale out the left nostril.

Step 11: Hold for 3 seconds.

Step 12: Inhale through your left nostril and repeat the cycle from the beginning.

Repeat for 3 to 7 cycles.

6-3-6-3 breathing

Step 1: Inhale through both nostrils to a count of 6.

Step 2: Hold the breath at the inhale for 3 seconds.

Step 3: Exhale for a count of 6.

Step 4: Hold the breath at the exhale for 3 seconds.

Step 5: Start again.

Repeat for 3 to 7 cycles.

Working through the layers

A cleanse or detox is a process that can involve a lot more than just your liver. It can affect your mental, physical, and spiritual bodies. To help you experience truly transformative health, start by releasing patterns that are no longer serving you.

Right now, take a moment to connect with your heart and check in with yourself. Use this time and space to help identify the old that is ready to be flushed out so that you can invite in transformational wellness. For some ideas of where to focus on while cleaning out the emotional layers, download our cleanse journal here: http://drheatherpaulson.com/bookresources/

Journaling is a space for reflecting and setting an intention for exactly what you want to release in your cleanse process. Often times, when we try to initiate new patterns, they don't stick because we have not completely flushed out the old. Once you identify the old patterns that are not serving your best health, and look at areas that might need attention in your physical and emotional body, it's time to make some juicy, feel-good, loving commitments to your transformation.

During your cleanse, I invite you to stop making commitments from a place of judgment, fear, or self-contempt. These commitments are not "shoulds" or "have-tos." These commitments come from a place of self-love and the desire for wholeness. For it is only when we come into being wholly ourselves that we experience true health. Here are some ideas of loving intentions you might like to make.

I will love my physical body during the cleanse.

Examples of where you might focus: moving 20 minutes a day, eating meals that are nourishing, eliminating caffeine.

I will love my emotional body during the cleanse.

Examples of where you might focus: journaling, practicing forgiveness, dedicating 5 minutes to self-care daily.

I will love my spiritual body during the cleanse.

Examples of where you might focus: meditating for 5 minutes a day, going to church/temple, reading a spiritual book, watching an inspiring movie, dedicating some time to a service project.

Relationship cleansing

During an emotional cleanse, ceremony and ritual can be an important practice to symbolize a shift or transition. As we get ready to enter a new phase of life, what are you ready to release? Is there something you are happy to leave behind with the pre-cleanse you?

Ceremony for emotional release

Creating a ceremony to let go of what is no longer serving you is a great way to move forward feeling light and bright. It helps you fully leave the past in the past.

One way you can do this is by writing down the people, places, and experiences you are ready to release. Light a fire in a contained fire-safe place. Place your notes with the names you wrote down into the fire. As it burns say, "I release you, I release you, I release you."

When the items are done burning, invite in the new experiences you are ready to receive.

Ceremony for physical release

Keep it simple. This isn't a complete closet clean-out or a hoarders intervention! If you need that, schedule it for after cleansing and let this be a jumping-off point.

To do a physical release, pick one or two items that are representative of where you are feeling stuck in your life. Fat clothes? Skinny clothes? Let them go now! You aren't either of those people any more. Old notes from school or a past job? Time to meet the recycle bin. Goals from the past? Tear them up. What didn't get done is past. What did get done can be celebrated. Either way, release the physical evidence to move forward cleanly.

Be fully present with where you are right now. Release the physical ties that keep you bound to the past.

Need more help?

Are you feeling like you might need more support in your detoxification or cleanse journey? I have created more resources for you.

Detoxing Home Chemicals Checklist: Overwhelmed with where to start removing toxins from your home? Grab this simple room-by-room checklist of what to eliminate and what to replace it with: http://drheatherpaulson.com/bookresources/

Cleanse Recipes: Need ideas of what to eat on your cleanse? Get three weeks of meals plans and recipes here: http://drheatherpaulson.com/bookresources/

Cleanse Community: Don't want to go it alone? Join our private Facebook group where you can post questions, ask for support, and connect with others on a similar journey:
https://www.facebook.com/groups/greatlifeplan/

CHAPTER 6:
THE POWER OF YOUR MIND

❋—❋—❋

Your mind is a powerful tool in healing. It is your healing space where you can connect with your body's innate wisdom and ability to heal. That means it's an essential part of living a *Cancer Proof* lifestyle.

In the coming chapter, you'll get everything you need to help you heal with the power of your mind, especially:

- the importance of mindset

- tools like affirmations, health visualizations, mantras and power words

- information on post-traumatic growth.

Does mindset make a difference?

Did you know that you already possess everything within you to be physically, emotionally, and spiritually well? You do! Your body wants you to be well. And using the power of your mind and thoughts is one step towards wellness.

It might seem kind of hokey to talk about mindset when

it comes to healing cancer. The truth is that mindset matters. And the research supports it. Dr. Lissa Rankin talks about how thoughts affect health in depth in her book *Mind Over Medicine*, where she focuses on the placebo and nocebo effects on health.

Placebo is when a positive effect is seen in a study group when giving a known *non-effector* (a substance already established as having no effect). Nocebo is an aggravation of symptoms or negative effect seen in the study group when giving a known non-effector.

Nocebo has been shown to impact death from surgeries, increase heart disease in women who thought they were going to get heart disease, and even to contribute to people dying when given a misdiagnosis of a deadly disease. One study looked specifically at patients who were believed to be terminal, and mistakenly informed that they had only a few months to live. The study subjects died in the predicted timeframe, even though they were mistakenly diagnosed with a disease that they didn't have. Even autopsy findings found no physiological reason for an early death.

Bottom line here is that our thoughts shape our reality. I love this zen quote from Ernest Holmes, because it rings so true… "Where your mind goes your energy flows."

From a physiological perspective, fear and stress trigger a slew of negative hormonal, inflammatory, and immune system effects. However, positive thoughts trigger a parasympathetic, or very calm state of being. In this state of calm, your body can rest, digest, and heal. Where do you want your energy to flow? Towards healing or illness?

Now, I'm not asking you to be a Pollyanna, or see the world unrealistically. Cancer sucks. I know that first hand. And there are studies supporting the idea that being overly optimistic is negative for your health too. However, could there be a middle space where positive intention, constructive thoughts, and becoming a statistical anomaly (as I like to call my patients) is born from a space of grounding and not illusion? I believe there is.

If you're not naturally optimistic, you might have to fake it until you make it. If you can't make it all the way to positive, being neutral might be more beneficial than being either optimistic or pessimistic.

Research has shown that thinking positively can:

- increase life span

- decrease depression

- reduce stress

- improve resilience

- reduce the risk of getting a cold

- increase psychological and physical wellness

- reduce the risk of cardiovascular death

- improve coping in times of stress and hardship.

Shifting self-talk

Positive self-talk is one of the most important areas to focus on when it comes to mindset. One way to think of positive self-talk is to not talk to yourself in a way that you would never talk to a friend or family member. Often, we can let our internal thoughts become so much meaner than anything we would ever say out loud to another person.

Let's practice shifting some negative thought patterns into positive ones. These are some examples that I hear in my office with patients who have or are recovering from cancer.

Negative Self-Talk	Alternative Positive Self-Talk
I am going to die from my cancer.	Today I am living and well.
This isn't going to work.	I can try to make this work.
It's too big of a change. I can't do it.	I'm willing to try to make a change. I'm going to try to make a change.

I'm too tired to get this done.	I will look at my priorities and see when I can get this done during my high energy time.
It's too complicated.	I have all the tools and support I need. If I can't figure it out, I can ask for help.
I've never eaten this kind of food.	I will take this diet change as an opportunity to explore new food and new choices.

And when all else fails, just add a "yet" to the end of your negative sentence.

I'm not a healthy person.	*I'm not healthy, yet.*
I don't eat healthy food.	*I don't eat healthy, yet.*
I'm not physically fit to do exercise.	*I'm not physically fit, yet.*

Alternatively, you can change your mindset passively. This might be a good place to start, if you're having trouble making a shift. One of the easiest ways to improve your sense of happiness and positivity is to watch an amusing comical movie or TV show. Studies have found that after watching a funny program, people had improved immune function. So, no excuses! The least you can do is change the channel to improve your health!

Get grateful!

Another way to create a more positive mindset is through gratitude practices. By thinking of or writing down what you are grateful for, you can change your life for the positive. When gratitude was looked at in a group of women with breast cancer, the study found that women with higher levels of self-reported gratitude experienced less stress, depression, and irritability. Other benefits of gratitude included feeling happy, increased post-traumatic growth, and having fewer symptoms of cancer.

Another study looked at women with breast cancer who participated in a six-week gratitude intervention, compared to a group of women with breast cancer who did not participate. The gratitude intervention meant spending 10 minutes, once a week, for six week, writing a letter to someone they were grateful for or who did something especially kind for them. The participants did not have to send the letter, just write the letter. The women who participated in the gratitude intervention had less fear of death, less fear of recurrence, and pursued meaningful goals.

In people without cancer, gratitude has been linked to greater happiness, life satisfaction or feeling fulfilled in their life, improved sense of wellbeing, and increased productivity.

A simple way to start integrating gratitude into your life is to keep a gratitude journal, sticky note, or memo on your smartphone. Every day, recognize three moments, people or experiences you are grateful for in your life. Studies have shown that the benefits of expressing gratitude are even greater when the events are noted daily, and when the experiences for which gratitude is expressed are smaller everyday happenings.

Post-traumatic growth

Changing post-traumatic stress to post-traumatic growth is another way in which mindset can impact your health. Cancer is a known event that causes post-traumatic stress in both cancer survivors, and their co-survivors or caregivers. But did you know that you can change post-traumatic stress into post-traumatic growth?

Post-traumatic growth is based on the idea that people can be changed, in a good way, by their struggles and hardships. This is represented in fairy tales, spiritual stories, and just about every feel-good movie out there. In fact, this is the journey that Joseph Campbell called "The Hero's Journey", which has since been the string tying together just about every popular story from Star Wars to the underdog winning the pennant race.

Research that looks at cancer as an event trigger of post-traumatic growth is on the rise. Some studies have revealed that 83% of breast cancer patients reported finding some benefit in their experience. In general, 60-

90% of individuals with cancer state that they believe they benefited in some way from their cancer experience. This isn't just true for cancer; all kinds of stressful or traumatic situations can trigger growth.

The most common positive outcomes from a cancer diagnosis included:

- enhanced interpersonal relationships

- greater appreciation for life

- sense of increased personal strength

- greater spirituality

- valued change in life priorities or life goals

- making positive health changes.

The benefits of a post-traumatic growth mindset can be improved mood, reduction in the stress hormone cortisol, increased immune function, and reduced pain. So we know it's desirable! But how do you go about shifting post-traumatic stress to post-traumatic growth? The answer is intentional engagement. You can engage intentionally in growth by starting to ask yourself some of life's deeper questions:

- What is life's worth?

- How do I uniquely contribute to the world?

- What is one time I showed more strength or

courage than I thought I had?

- What do I consider the most valuable things in life?

Pure existence is an amazing act. Focus on the wonder of life.

Visualization for better health

Did you know your brain is so powerful that just thinking about doing physical exercise can change your muscle and brain structure? A study done by the Cleveland Clinic showed that people who visualized contracting the abductor muscles in their thighs had a 35% increase in muscle strength compared to those who did not visualize leg contractions.

Could this apply to cancer? What if you applied this technique to natural killer cells? Or immune function? I had one patient who would visualize chemotherapy melting away his tumors. If you are preventing cancer, you can visualize your continued good health. If you are a cancer survivor recovering from treatments, you can visualize yourself strong, healthy, and active. Research studies show that this actually could increase your natural killer cell counts.

Other studies have looked at the power of visualizing peaceful scenes while listening to relaxing music. It was found that people undergoing cancer treatment who practiced these therapies had reduced nausea from chemotherapy, less anxiety, a more positive mood, increased natural killer cells, reduced cortisol levels; overall, they felt better. It was as simple as listening to two guided imagery audio tracts while receiving their chemotherapy.

Some ways to put visualization into practice is to use a guided imagery meditation, listen to affirmations, or record your own affirmations.

Affirmations

Positive affirmations can be used to help access your inner strength and coping skills. Some examples of positive affirmations for cancer include:

I am so happy to be living a long and healthy life.

I am so grateful for a full recovery and a healthy life.

I am healthy and happy.

I live a life of good health, happiness, joy, and meaning.

Feel free to borrow these as a starting point, but do also explore your own. The most meaningful affirmations are the ones you create for yourself. To create your own affirmations:

- Keep it simple.

- Affirm the feeling or outcome that you want to have.

- Make sure your affirmations are written in a positive form. (For example: instead of saying "I am not sick", it would be preferable to state, "I am completely free of illness.")

- Write your affirmations as if it has already occurred and you are speaking in the present tense.

Mantras

Mantras are slightly different to affirmations. Some people like them better because they can be simpler. A mantra is any saying, song, statement, or slogan repeated over and over. I have seen some of my patients use songs like "Fight Song" as their mantra. A mantra can also be as simple as repeating Om, Amen, or a piece of spiritual scripture.

No matter what kind of mantra you choose, make it a powerful daily practice that helps connect you to the inner strength you have to move forward in a *Cancer Proof* life.

Whatever you choose to do to help visualize your health, make sure it's something you can stick with, feels personal to you, and doesn't feel fake. Most importantly, in those moments when you are feeling icky, sad, or angry, make sure you have a safe space to get those negative emotions out without judgment or placating them with overly positive statements. It's okay to have down moments too. Just remember that in order to be your most powerful, healthy self, your thoughts and words have implications on your overall health that cannot be underestimated.

CHAPTER 7:
HEALING MEDITATIONS

❋—❋—❋

Whatever you've been told about meditation, let's take this chapter to bust some myths and set you on a path to a calmer journey through cancer.

We'll explore:

- the power of meditation on cancer cells and your overall health

- specific practices like walking, sitting, breathing, guided, quiet

- inner smile meditation and prayer.

Hype or healing?

You might have noticed all the mindfulness and meditation info popping up all over the place! Even *Cosmopolitan* magazine has gotten into the craze, and I wouldn't define Cosmo as a particularly spiritually enlightened read for the most part! Beyond magazines, corporations like Google are teaching meditation and mindfulness to improve work productivity and satisfaction. Is it all hype or is there something worth paying attention? Here we'll take a look at the literature so you can decide for yourself.

Now, before we get started and in case you're wondering if meditation is part of a specific religion, let me put that to rest for you. It's not part of any particular religion or religious practice. However, all the major religions discuss the use of meditation in their spiritual texts including the Bible, Torah, Yoga Sutras, Bhagavad Gita, and the Koran.

With that question answered, let's start by going through some of the recent meditation research. The good news is that there is a lot of medical literature that highlights whether meditation works, how it works, and when it works. When it comes to the conditions meditation can treat, it's all over the map!

How meditation works

Evidence suggests that mindfulness practices are associated with neuroplastic changes in the anterior cingulate cortex, insula, temporo-parietal junction, fronto-limbic network, and default mode network structures. What does that mean in non-neuroscientist speak? Meditation can improve the areas of the brain that are associated with:

- focus

- body awareness

- emotional regulation

- re-evaluation

- flexible self concept

- enhanced self-regulation.

Functional and structural neuroimaging studies, or taking pictures of brain activity, have begun to explore the neuroscientific processes underlying these areas of the brain and the impact meditation is having on the brain.

Research shows that as little as 27 minutes of meditation practice per day increases gray matter. (When gray matter shrinks with age, it can lead to dementia among other conditions.) Participants that meditated for 27 minutes also had a reduction in the amygdala, or the area of the brain associated with fear, panic, and the sympathetic fight-or-flight response. The participants also noticed an increase in self-awareness, compassion, and introspection.

Some physiological benefits of meditation include a reduction in the stress hormone cortisol, reduced inflammation as expressed through interleukin-6. IL-6 is particularly interesting in cancer care, because when it is elevated, it can directly influence cancer growth and protection of metastatic cancer cells.

If you're looking for a more positive mood, look no

further than meditation. It has been shown to increase feel-good neurotransmitters like serotonin, dopamine, and melatonin. One benefit of increasing the latter is that proper melatonin levels have been shown to be protective against cancer cells and might even reduce risk of recurrence. In addition to increasing the happy brain chemicals, meditation can reduce the not so-happy-brain chemicals like noradrenaline.

Meditation can help decrease pain and reduce perceived fatigue. This could be because it increases beta-endorphins and arginine vasopressin.

Meditation benefits

Here is a list of the specific conditions that can benefit from meditation.

- **Inflammation:** Reduced COX-2 expression, IL-6, and NF-kappa B. Can also reduce nerve inflammation.

- **Pain:** Significant reduction in lower back pain. Lower pain sensitivity and increased analgesic effects experienced during mindful states. All it takes is 20 minutes for three days.

- **Addiction to smoking, food, or alcohol:** Improved self-control, smoking reduction up to 60%, less relapse.

- **Infection:** Reduced risk of viral infection, and

missed days from work due to infection and shortened duration of viral illness. Even when a virus was present in the bloodstream according to a blood test, those who meditated were less likely to show any signs or symptoms of illness.

- **Blood sugar:** Improved insulin response.

- **Blood pressure:** Reduced systolic and diastolic blood pressure readings, reduced heart rate.

- **Depression:** Helps prevent depression relapse, improves depressive symptoms.

- **Anxiety:** Reduced anxiety symptoms by 22%, after just 20 minutes of meditation.

- **Insomnia:** Improved sleep quality, reduced daytime impairments from too little sleep.

- **Other:** Reduced chronic occupational stress, enhanced empathy, reduced mistakes.

Further to the general health benefits, in patients undergoing treatment for cancer, meditation can reduce side effects of treatments, improve concentration and mood, increase immune function, and decrease anxiety and depression.

Meditation techniques to try

There are many ways to engage in meditation and it doesn't have to be hard or inaccessible. You don't have to be sitting on a cushion chanting in a cave somewhere to meditate successfully. In fact, you don't have to be sitting or chanting at all. First comes mindfulness, a type of meditation practice that requires no changes to your current routine. Then, we have techniques like walking meditation, and of course sitting in a meditative state. The most important part to remember is that this is only going to feel good when you find a practice that works for you.

Guided meditation

If you're unsure about whether you'll be able to sit in silence or worried about doing meditation "correctly", guided meditation can be a great place to start. Guided meditation is defined as a state of relaxed concentration being guided by a teacher, religious guide, audio recording, or even your own voice being played back to yourself.

My favorite guided meditation is the Meditation on Twin Hearts guided by Master Choa Kok Sui. This particular guided meditation has been indicated in a study to create the same brain waves as a monk who has been meditating for 20 years in a monastery in participants who are not monks.

In the research, subjects doing the Twin Hearts meditation also experienced immediately improved happiness, improved empathy, decreased anxiety, and faster reaction times. The longer someone practices the

Meditation on Twin Hearts, the greater the gamma waves in their brain, which leads to improved emotional regulation and attention. Lastly, it increased serum melatonin by more than 300% on the levels prior to meditation.

Mindfulness

Mindfulness meditation is the state of being conscious or aware of something. To put mindfulness into practice, you constantly and consistently focus on the present moment. As an extension to this practice of coming back to the present moment, you may also calmly acknowledge and accept your feelings, thoughts, and the sensations in your physical body.

In one of my favorite documentaries called "How to Cook Your Life", a zen priest describes cooking as the ultimate practice in mindfulness. From coming into the present moment with the sensation of kneading bread, or hearing a kettle come to the boil, daily activities can be a point of connecting with mindfulness. Some of my patients find it easy to bring mindfulness to a cup of tea, taking a walk, or washing the dishes. Mindfulness isn't about *what* you are doing; it's about *how* you are present while you are doing it.

Walking

Using the simplicity of walking as a form of meditation is a common zen practice. It is recommended to do 10 minutes of walking meditation daily. Jon Kabat-Zinn in the book *Mindfulness Meditation in Everyday Life* suggests doing a walking meditation by finding a location where you can walk back and forth 10 to 15 paces. This space can be indoors or outdoors.

Once you have found a location, start by walking 10 to 15 steps, then pause and breathe. When you are ready and done pausing, turn around and walk the 10 to 15 steps back to where you started, retracing your path. Continue repeating this sequence.

Once you are comfortable with the walk and pace, you can add some words or awareness to the walk by noticing each part of walking. You can say: *I am lifting my foot. I am moving my foot forward. I am placing my foot on the floor heel first. I am shifting my weight. I am lifting the heel of the back foot. My toes are touching the ground. I am lifting my back foot completely off the floor. My foot is swinging forward. My foot is lowering. My foot is contacting the ground heel first. My weight is shifting. My body is moving forward.*

You can also move your attention to your breath, your arms, your shoulders, or any other bodily sensation. If your mind begins to wander, gently bring your attention back to the sensations and movements.

Sitting or concentration meditation

Once you move into sitting, concentration, or Dhyana meditation, you are dropping the mindfulness of physical sensations. This type of mediation is built on the experience of nothingness. You are quieting all the senses in your body and thoughts in your mind. If you need to point your focus towards something, you can point it towards connecting with God or feeling the love that surrounds you.

To experience this type of meditation:

- Sit comfortably in a quiet spot.

- Set a timer for 5 to 10 minutes. Even two minutes just to start.

- Relax your eyelids and your jaw.

- Direct your attention to an area of focus; one example would be to focus on the gap between your inhale and exhale of breath.

- As distracting thoughts pop into your mind, instead of focusing on them, let them go and refocus on the breath.

This type of meditation should be free of effort. If you are putting in effort to empty the mind, you are missing some of the meditative benefits. By raising your awareness above the physical and detaching from sensations and thoughts, you are free to connect with the bliss state that can be experienced through meditation.

Breathing or Pranayama

Noticing the breath is one of the simplest ways to start a

meditation or relaxation practice. You can become aware of how the breath moves in and out of the nostrils, how the breath is filling the lungs, the pause in between inhaling and exhaling. You can do this sitting or standing.

This is a practice that shows benefits for reducing a stressed state when done for as little as two minutes, so having enough time in the day can't be an excuse for not meditating!

There are other breathing practices that help clear certain energy bodies. We went through one such breathing exercise, alternate nostril breathing, in Chapter 6: Detox. There are other types of breathing exercise that can be used for concentrating the mind: pranic breathing, lion breath, the breath of fire, ocean breath, and turtle breathing. Each one of these practices benefits different areas of the energetic anatomy.

If you currently have cancer, I recommend sticking to the breathing exercises outlined in Chapter 5 and pranic breathing. Those are the safest breathing practice for most people. Pranic breathing, as taught by Master Stephen Co, can be experienced by following these steps:

- Sit on the edge of a chair or sofa, keeping your back straight.

- Place your thumbs on your belly button, allowing your fingers to lay across the lower abdomen.

- Place your tongue to the roof of your mouth, at the ridge just behind the hard palate.

- Exhale through your mouth until your lungs are completely empty.

- Inhale for a count 3, hold for 1 second at the top of the breath, exhale for a count of 3, hold for 1 second at the bottom of the exhale.

- Start the inhalation cycle over again.

As your lung capacity improves, you may choose to extend the rhythm to inhaling for 6, holding for 3 seconds, exhaling for 6. Another rhythm is to inhale for 7, hold for 4 seconds, exhale for 7. You can find many different rhythms in qi gong, yoga, and martial art practices.

The next safest breathing technique would be the ocean breath. The ocean breath is known for calming the mind. It can be experienced by doing this:

- With your lips closed, start breathing in and out of your nose.

- Place your tongue to the roof of your palate.

- As you exhale out your nose, relax the throat.

- Allow the exhaled breath to make a noise while coming through the throat and nose, similar to the noise of an ocean wave crashing on the beach.

The turtle breath can be another way to clear the mind, and tap into a sense of calm and peace. To experience turtle breathing, here's what you do:

- Place your tongue to the roof of your mouth, at the ridge where the hard and soft palate come together.

- Fully exhale and empty your lungs as completely as possible.

- Inhale through your nose while lifting your chin up to the sky, dipping your head backwards.

- As you exhale through your slightly open mouth, bring your chin to your chest.

- Repeat the inhale and exhale cycle seven times.

The lion breath and breath of fire may be too stimulating for people with cancer or recovering from cancer. If you are interested in incorporating these breathing techniques, please consult a yoga teacher, pranic healer, or doctor to see if they are okay for you.

If you think it would be easier to watch a video of any of these breathing techniques, we have examples at: http://drheatherpaulson.com/bookresources/

The overarching benefits of breathing practices include:

- relaxation

- clearing the energy body

- improving oxygenation of the blood and tissue

- calming the nervous system

- relieving anxiety

- providing headache relief

- increasing immune function

- reducing blood pressure

- increasing energy levels

- relaxing the muscles

- decreasing feelings of stress and overwhelm

- improving lung health.

Metta or loving kindness meditation

The use of Metta meditation is something that studies have shown measurably increases compassion and empathy. If you feel like this is something you need to cultivate in your life, the Metta meditation is a great place to start. The Metta meditation is done by reciting the following:

May I be happy. May I be well. May I be safe. May I be peaceful and at ease.

After you let these blessings sink in, allow yourself to visualize someone you love. Then say:

May you be happy. May you be well. May you be safe. May you be peaceful and at ease.

Continue repeating this for as many people, animals, and beings with whom you want to share these blessings. When you are ready to move on, bring to mind someone you have a grievance with or have a hard time understanding. Then say:

May you be happy. May you be well. May you be safe. May you be peaceful and at ease.

If you notice any feelings or resentment, anger, sadness, or grief rise up while doing this meditation, you can go back to the first step and apply loving acceptance to yourself and your own thoughts.

Prayer

Praying is defined as a solemn request for help or expression of thanks addressed to God or an object of worship. Prayer is used as a way to create a connection, conversation, or communion with God. Prayer can take many forms depending on what spiritual tradition you are practicing.

Where meditation and prayer cross over is in the point of

silence. When you sit in prayer silently, connecting with God, and waiting for inspiration to come through, this is a practice of meditation.

Participating in prayer can:

- improve self-control

- reduce feelings of anger

- help us become more forgiving of those for whom we pray

- increase feelings of trust and unity

- reduce feelings of stress

- facilitate a radical remission.

Studies have shown that people receiving prayers in a blinded way (so they don't know someone is praying for them) have improved outcomes compared to those who did not have prayers. This has also been shown in infertility studies, wound healing studies, and other health conditions to improve the efficacy of treatments and improve the outcomes.

Labyrinth

Using a walking meditation like a labyrinth can be a great tool for improving our connection to the inner voice that knows the direction our life needs to take. This inner voice might be considered God, your intuition, or simply a sense of inner knowing. No matter what you call this voice, tuning in and cultivating awareness allows you to live life in the flow with your highest calling.

If you are seeking answers, try walking a labyrinth as a type of prayer. I like the labyrinth as a tool to discover my inner thoughts on the bigger questions, or to let go of belief patterns or emotions that are holding me back from experiencing my best life.

Steps to utilizing a labyrinth:

- Think of or write down a problem or question that you need help resolving. If you prefer to release a thought, person, or emotion, bring it to mind or write it down.

- Walk into the labyrinth starting at the entrance and walking clockwise. Keep your thought, prayer, or question in your mind as you walk one foot in front of the other.

- If you get distracted or find your mind wandering, go back to your thought or prayer. Inhale, exhale, focus on your breathing, or on your foot striking the ground: heel, ball, toe, lift.

- Make sure you walk the labyrinth at your own pace. Everyone will have a different speed or rhythm that is needed to feel grounded, connected, and present.

- Once you reach the middle, take as much time as you need to release your question, thought, or prayer. You might find yourself sitting in meditation for several minutes to several hours.

- Exit the labyrinth in a counterclockwise fashion. Keep the mind open and receptive. You might have answers or release come to you during this part of the walk. However, it can take days or months to see the results of your labyrinth walk.

- Stay open and receptive. Listen closely to hear the whispers of your soul or God.

That's it! If you don't have a walking labyrinth near you, you can use a finger labyrinth. It is a great seated meditation that can be used anywhere.

Downsides

So all of this sounds great, but are there downsides to meditation and mindfulness? Yes, there can be. It is common, as we start quieting the mind through meditation and come into a mindful state, that repressed emotions, old experiences, and past tendencies come to the surface. These negative emotions arise to be healed and transformed. If it is too much to do on your own, seek out a local meditation instructor, pranic healer, or counselor to help resolve the thoughts and emotions coming up.

Now that we have covered the many benefits of

meditation, different types of meditation, and how to incorporate meditation into your life, the next step is up to you. Reflect on how you'll start implementing a meditation practice into your life.

If you're looking for a guided meditation, you can enjoy this one that I recorded specifically for healing: http://drheatherpaulson.com/bookresources/

CHAPTER 8:
TROUBLESHOOTING AND
GOING DEEPER

❋—❋—❋

As we approach the end of our *Cancer Proof* journey together in this book, you may wonder what to do if none of this works. If you have noticed meaningful change, you might be craving a deeper look into what this all means. And there is so much more than a physical illness.

In this chapter, we'll explore:

- the soul of healing

- illness as a vehicle for transformation

- the power of prayer

- visiting sacred spaces, healing temples, sacred sites

- forgiveness and disease.

Turning inward

Health is not just an external journey. To be truly

healthy, you must dedicate time to turning inwards. In a traditional sense, the word *healing* simply means to return to wholeness. This is a time to acknowledge the many forms of health and healing. Sometimes the most magical way to return to wholeness is to tap into the spiritual side of health.

Returning to wholeness or health doesn't always mean "conquering", "fighting" or "winning" against a disease. Sometimes a return to wholeness means releasing our physical body this round and getting ready to see what is on the other side of this life. I was recently reminded of this when someone posted on social media about a loved one dying of cancer. Immediately, I returned to that young woman who sat down next to her dad while he took his last breath, wondering... *Where did all the doctors go? Why is nobody here to birth him into the next phase of his soul?*

To those of you reading this book who will inevitably let go of a loved one or your own body due to the effects of cancer, I would like to dedicate this chapter to you. You are not alone. There are so many of us who have walked this journey and know the heartache as well as the freedom associated with this stage of illness.

This is not a time to let go of natural therapies. They can be so helpful for pain management with clear cognition, for gentle exits, and powerful connections. They might not "cure" you, but they could give you more quality time with those you love. And isn't that really what's important about living this life? Connection.

As a cancer co-survivor, I have been that person clinging to connection and refusing to leave my husband in the hospital at closing time. Sleeping on a pullout bed. Holding his hand. It was a deeply transformational and life-changing time of our lives. He is alive and well now, but in those dark moments it felt like he was only connected to life by a teeny tiny thread.

I watched my dad release his physical body through cancer. In the midst of watching his body shut down were some of the most beautiful conversations and moments of life I have ever been blessed to witness. Rivaled only by the beauty of being part of a birthing team for a new soul entering this world is being one of the gifted few that get to sit with someone transitioning their soul into the next phase through physical death.

Now as a cancer doctor, it's important to me that we go to the dark sides of cancer care and talk about them, recognize them, and bring awareness to the shadows. Bringing awareness doesn't mean bringing light. Sometimes the shadows are dark and sad and scary. But that is all part of the human experience, not having to bring light to the shadows.

There is always hope. It's not the kind of hope that people talk about when they are trying to cheer you up about your disease and help you overcome it, fight it, beat it. Yet there is always hope that you can find a

greater sense of peace in the brevity of life. There is hope
that you will connect with Spirit, the Creator, the Divine,
whatever God is to you. There is hope that you will taste
the blips of time full of joy and bliss. There is hope that
death can be the ultimate yoga or union with the Soul -
even though it can be challenging and even painful to
disconnect the physical body from the spiritual soul.

The soul of illness and the soul of healing are such
personal parts of the human journey. Only you can define
what it is that your Soul is trying to gain from this
process, this illness, this journey. Sometimes, you will
never know in this lifetime the meaning of an illness. I
truly believe that it was part of my dad's soul contract to
die from cancer. His death from cancer was a pivotal
piece in transforming my path from being dedicated to
healing the planet to being focused on healing humans.
Years after his death while I was doing my residency in
oncology, I was hit by the enormity of the ripple effect
of my father's death. And now, when I walk into my
clinic named in his honor, with his picture at the entry
way, I'm reminded of the healing power and pain of
cancer.

Some of my patients go as far to say *thank you* to my
dad's picture as they read the mission and values of The
Paulson Center. Just today, a patient said to me, "I was
so touched by your story of how you got into cancer care.
I think your dad's death was a way for God to put you on
this path so you could help me today."

Did he know this ripple effect would happen? Absolutely not! Am I grateful for the traumatic growth experiences of my dad and my husband having cancer? Absolutely yes.

That is the more positive side of the soul of illness. But what about the negative? In my dad's journey with cancer, I can easily identify areas of his life where unresolved emotional pains, repressed emotions, and lack of self-care were a part of his illness forming. What were his life lessons from the experience of cancer? I wish I could go back and ask him this question. But no matter what he answered, it would not and could not impact your soul of illness, as this is unique to each individual. As unique as your genetic information.

The soul of illness is often a point of separation. When you are separated from the Soul, when your energy body is congested or blocked, this is the original initiation and soul of illness. These blockages can be caused by negative emotions, past wrongs that we have done to others, negative thoughts, and lessons requested by Spirit when entering the planet.

To learn the Soul of your illness and the deeper connection of your life, you can explore questions like: *Why am I here? What is my purpose? What unique gifts do I bring to the planet?*

You can also reflect on grievances. Reflecting on grievances is a way to release the past and move into the future clean and clear. We are all in the process of evolving and growing. In this process of being human, we have been hurt by others, but if we look at things fairly, it is also likely that we have incidentally hurt others too. To examine this deeper, you might ask yourself questions like: *Who have I not forgiven? Who do I need to receive forgiveness from? Where have I done things inappropriately because I didn't know any better at that time of my life? Why have I called in this injury or illness?*

Truthfully, there aren't always clear answers to these questions, and that is okay. The value isn't in the answers. It's in the act of contemplation. Sometimes we will never know the answers to these questions, in the same way my dad never knew the positive ripple effect of his cancer.

According to many spiritual healing traditions, the soul of illness can often come down to anger, resentment, lack of forgiveness, and negative karma. This isn't brought up for you to beat yourself up. I'm mentioning it here to bring it to your attention because there is *something you can do about it*. You can still commit acts of forgiveness, you can always improve positive karma through acts of service, and you can continue do the inner work necessary to resolve anger, resentment, and negative emotions.

Sometimes we block these opportunities to turn inwards and connect with Spirit. One of my great teachers, a

Cherokee medicine man, wisely says, "Pay attention to the moments where you are blocked from connecting with the Creator. Whatever comes up and blocks you from connecting — an email, phone call, errand, social media post — whatever it is, that is where you need to look deeper. That is where you can ask yourself: *Why am I allowing this disconnection? What am I receiving from this distraction?* Start there, and everything else will become clearer."

Forgiveness, releasing the past, and opening up to vibrancy and love

I first came across the idea of forgiveness being linked to cancer while talking to a Mauian Kahuna, or medicine man. I was studying his movements as he sorted through herbs to make healing teas. He was "talking story" with me, as the say in Maui, and sharing with me how important our thoughts are when making medicine, a concept overlooked in large manufacturing plants. He said that the energy we put into the medicine is the energy our patients experience from the medicine. Put in fear, anger, resentment and people will not heal. Put in love, forgiveness, and hope and people will get better.

This Kahuna then blessed me with the opportunity to ask a question. As someone continually on the search for the best way to heal cancer, I asked, "In your tradition, what is the cause of cancer?" I was curious because the way he viewed the body wasn't about cytokines, inflammatory markers, or immune function. He viewed the body as a divine instrument provided by Ka, the Hawaiian word for God.

The Kahuna's answer was quick and to the point. He answered without a pause, "Lack of forgiveness. That is the true cause of cancer. Anger, resentment, hurt. That is what makes cancer cells."

It is with this understanding that I have taken in this information, and share with you these simple forgiveness practices.

In the Mauian tradition, there is a forgiveness practice known as ho'oponopono, a prayer that has been passed on from Kahuna to Kahuna for generations. Ho'oponopono is defined in the Hawaiian dictionary as "mental cleansing: family conferences in which relationships were set right through prayer, discussion, confession, repentance, and mutual restitution and forgiveness." It is the idea that all relations are connected. And that we have to make right this connection in order to be well.

While the ceremony is sacred, and can be experienced with a Kahuna in the Hawaiian and Polynesian Islands, a westernized version has been released to the public.

Ho'oponopono practice

Do this practice to make right with all your relations and free up energy for other parts of your life.

1. Bring to mind anyone with whom you do not feel total alignment or support.

2. In your mind's eye, construct a small stage below you.

3. Imagine an infinite source of love and healing flowing from a source above the top of your head (from your Higher Self, God, or whatever you connect with). Imagine opening up the top of your head, and letting the source of love and healing flow down inside your body, filling up the body, and overflowing from your heart to heal the person on the stage.

4. Say to the person: *I am sorry, Please forgive me. I love you. Thank you.*

5. When the healing is complete, have a discussion with the person and forgive them, and have them forgive you.

6. Next, let go of the person, and see them floating away. As they do, cut the cord that connects the two of you (if appropriate). If you are healing in a current primary relationship, then assimilate the person inside you.

7. Do this with every person in your life with whom you are incomplete, or not aligned. The final test is: *Can you see the person or think of them without feeling any negative emotions?* If you do

feel negative emotions, do the ho'oponopono process again.

This is one of the many forms of forgiveness practice you could try, but there are many throughout the world.

If ho'oponopono does not resonate with you, offer a prayer that speaks to your spiritual practice. Forgiveness is a common thread between all spiritual teachings whether you are Christian, Muslim, Hindu, Buddhist, or Jewish. Some other traditional prayers of forgiveness include:

- forgiveness meditation

- the Prayer of Saint Francis

- Buddhist Metta meditation (as in Chapter 7: Healing Meditations)

- "I hereby forgive" Jewish bedtime prayer

While doing any forgiveness practice, keep in mind that forgiveness is for you. It releases *you* from the chains of a negative thought or person. A forgiveness practice is an inner practice. You might still have to stand up for yourself or protect yourself outwardly, but inwardly you forgive.

Forgiveness meditation of Master Choa Kok Sui

1. Put your hands together in prayer position at the heart.

2. Visualize in front of you the person who you wish to forgive.

3. Say to the person, "The child of God within me recognizes the child of God within you."

4. Visualize the face of the person slowly fading into a ball of brilliant light. Greet this being of light again.

5. Say to this person: "We are all children of God. We are all in the process of evolving. Evolution involves time, process, and lots of mistakes. I had my share of mistakes, and learned from them. So can you. I wish you the same. God's peace and love be with me. God's peace and love be with you. You are completely forgiven. May you be blessed with inner peace and inner healing. May you be blessed with spiritual transformation and spiritual maturity. God's blessings be with you. May you grow spiritually and evolve. Namaste. You are completely forgiven. Go in peace. I completely release you. Go in peace. Cut, cut, cut! I release you. I release you. I release you."

Forgiveness meditation by Desmond Tutu

1. Close your eyes and follow your breath. When you feel centered, imagine yourself in a safe place.

2. In the center of your safe space is a box with

many drawers. The drawers are labeled. The inscriptions show hurts you have yet to forgive.

3. Choose a drawer and open it. Rolled or folded or crumpled up inside it are all the thoughts and feelings the incident evokes.

4. You can choose to empty out this drawer. Bring your hurt into the light and examine it. Unfold the resentment you have felt and set it aside. Smooth out the ache and let it drift up into the sunlight and disappear. If any feeling seems too big or too unbearable, set it aside to look at later.

5. When the drawer is empty, sit for a moment with it on your lap. Then remove the label from this drawer.

6. As the label comes off, you will see the drawer turn to sand. The wind will sweep it away. You don't need it anymore. There will be no space left for that hurt in the box. That space is not needed anymore.

7. If there are more drawers still to be emptied, you can repeat this meditation now or later.

Prayer of Saint Francis

Lord, make me an instrument of thy peace.

Where there is hatred, let me sow love;

Where there is injury, pardon;

Where there is doubt, faith;

Where there is darkness, light;

Where there is sadness, joy.

O divine Master, grant that I may not so much seek

To be consoled as to console,

To be understood as to understand,

To be loved as to love;

For it is in giving that we receive;

It is in pardoning that we are pardoned;

And it's in dying that we are born to eternal life.

Amen.

Benefits of inner forgiveness

Once you have fully released a person, your body will feel lighter. You may notice your mood lifting too. Occasionally, just by doing a forgiveness practice, you will notice your relationships shifting and becoming filled with more joy and love.

As we let go of the past, we make room for the present. As we release resentment, anger, and hurt, we make room for joy, love, and happiness. Give yourself the gift of forgiveness at least once a month.

Sacred spaces of healing

There are many phenomena that our current realms of science cannot explain and one of these is healing within the walls of sacred spaces. While on a trip to France, I was gifted with the opportunity to visit Lourdes. Although I am not a practicing Catholic, the sanctity of this space was clear as soon as we stepped foot onto the grounds.

I was totally blown away by the number of people who had traveled from all over the world to experience the healing power of the water of Lourdes. The hospitals there transport their occupants to the waters several times a day. There are many stories of miraculous healing and transformation. It is truly a beautiful thing to witness and participate in the blessings, services, and healing taking place at Lourdes.

There are many healing sites like this throughout the world: Brazil, Maui, Peru, the American plains and desert, Egypt, Israel, Bali, India, Tibet, Bhutan, Sedona. Every continent has their sacred healing sites. It might seem weird that a doctor steeped in Western medical science would talk about sacred healing sites. Over the years, I have seen so many instances of healing that are completely missed by focusing on blood work and scans alone. They are intangible, indescribable.

I wish that everyone could experience the unique level

of transformation and healing that can only happen when you visit holy and sacred sites. It is hard to explain in writing the peace that comes from these sites. No matter what religion or spiritual tradition you practice, it is likely that you have a sacred site that calls your name. If not a religious center, it might be a picture of an outdoor space, mountain range, or ocean. These natural formations can carry the energy of healing.

Something you should know if you choose to go on a spiritual healing pilgrimage that sometimes I tend to forget... Part of the healing and transformation happens in the attempt alone. In fact, some of the deepest transformation and healing can happen during the journey to the site. Be gentle with yourself while you travel. If obstacles come up, view them with curiosity and introspection.

I would like to close with a meditative prayer offered by the great teacher Master Choa Kok Sui.

I AM the Soul.

I AM not the body.

I AM not the emotion.

I AM not the thought.

I Am not the mind.

I AM the Soul.

I AM a spiritual being of Divine Intelligence, Divine Love, Divine Power.

I AM one with my Higher Soul.

I AM THAT I AM.

I AM one with the Divine Spark within me.

I AM a child of God.

I AM connected with God.

I AM one with God.

I AM one with All.

May you find your path to reconnection with wholeness. May you be divinely blessed with health, healing, joy, and wholeness. Thank you for sharing this journey with me.

CLOSING AND NEW BEGINNINGS

❋—❋—❋

Now, the *Cancer Proof* journey begins...

I know a lot of information was covered in this book and you might still be wondering...

- How exactly does this apply to me?

- How can I individualize my health plan?

- Are there certain supplements I should be taking?

- How can I travel to some of those spiritually healing locations?

Or maybe you have a totally different question that I haven't even covered yet. That's why this book is just a jumping-off point for our conversation together. I'm here to support you through this journey step by step.

If you would like to schedule a time to review your individual questions and have a unique plan formulated just for you, please visit www.drheatherpaulson.com and click on the "Schedule Now" button or call the office at

480-939-3589.

If you are interested in experiencing a healing retreat, a spiritual healing center of the world, or just taking some time for resetting self-care practices, you can be placed on our retreat waitlist here:
http://drheatherpaulson.com/bookresources/

We can also continue this conversation in the private Facebook group at
https://www.facebook.com/groups/greatlifeplan/

Don't forget to check out the resources page for extra videos, guides, and downloads to support the information you learned in this book. The *Cancer Proof* resource page is:
http://drheatherpaulson.com/bookresources/

No matter how we stay connected, I'm looking forward to supporting your next leg of the journey.

To Your Health!

Dr. Heather Paulson

ACKNOWLEDGEMENTS

——*

Even though there is only one name as the author, it is not a solitary process to write a book! Many people went into creating this healing and transformation.

With gratitude for his enduring support, grocery shopping, and cheering me on, I'd like to thank my husband Phil. If our journey together didn't include the wonder of combining naturopathic care with chemotherapy, this book would never exist. Countless people are impacted by your story, dedication, and making sure our healing clinic is one that is comfortable for everyone – even those who, like you, don't like doctors. It is life-changing for so many people.

I would also like to thank every patient who has taught me along the way. Each one of you has shaped the physician that I have become. While writing, I imagined you sitting across the table, guiding me on what to talk about and how to help you crack a smile. Without you, this book would be a boring pile of research papers.

I am grateful for my family who edited, read, and gave feedback on this book. Or just cheered me on when my fingers were going numb from typing. Thanks Mom,

Aunt Diane, and Uncle Gary. I couldn't have done it without you.

I would like to also acknowledge Alicia, Rhonda, and Stephania. You were there for me when Phil was going through chemo, through medical school, residency, hosting my first retreat, and forming a business. You always see me as something greater than I can possibly see myself. Thank you for holding the vision of what can be, so my dad's story can help transform others.

I also acknowledge my teachers Master Stephen Co and Grand Master Choa Kok Sui for guiding my spiritual path. You have opened me up to the depth and beauty of healing with prana, forgiveness, meditation, and breathing. The gifts of pranic healing ripple in countless way through out my life and the lives of my patients.

And to the countless other people who have showed up in support: Kris Emery, Richard Taubinger, Razi Berry, Jennifer Havens, Shana Boyer, Keith and Lesley McCloghrie, Julie Kenkel, Rene Goades-Caves, Murchi Javelosa, Brian Pry, Lois Nicholls, Duane and Susan Anderson, Jeff Potts, Hillary Barrese, Sandy and Jim Millsap, Natalie MacNeil, Courtney Johnston, Yasmine Khater, Laura Ribas, Holly Bertone.

ABOUT THE AUTHOR

※ — ※ — ※

D r. Heather Paulson is a teacher, author, lecturer, researcher, and physician in the field of integrative and naturopathic oncology. Her specialized area of practice focuses on utilizing integrative, natural, and naturopathic therapies to support people impacted by cancer. She lectures to international audiences on the many aspects of integrative, functional, and naturopathic oncology.

As adjunct faculty at the Southwest College of Naturopathic Medicine, Dr. Heather Paulson teaches oncology and hematology. In this role, she is also co-writing the Textbook of Naturopathic and Integrative Oncology.

In addition to teaching, Heather continues The Paulson Center for Integrative Healing. A center that includes naturopaths, acupuncturists, counselors, massage therapists, aestheticians, nutritionists, and energy workers coming together to support people diagnosed with cancer.

She has been featured on local news programs Sonoran Living and Your Health A-Z as guest speaker on natural cancer care. She has also published several oncology-based articles in NDNR and Natural Medicine Journal. Dr. Heather Paulson has also been a featured abstract presenter at the Society for Integrative Oncology.

FURTHER READING

✳—✳—✳

The following are studies, resources and references used throughout this book. You can also find more *Cancer Proof* resources on the website at:
http://drheatherpaulson.com/bookresources/

Books

The Cancer-Fighting Kitchen by Rebecca Katz

The Survivor's Handbook: Eating Right for Cancer Survival by Dr. Neal Bernard

Anticancer: A New Way of Life by David Servan-Schreiber

Food Rules by Michael Pollan

The Power of Rest: Why Sleep Alone Is Not Enough by Matthew Edlund

Take a Nap! Change Your Life by Mark Ehrman and Sara Mednick

Essentialism: The Disciplined Pursuit of Less by Greg McKeown

Websites

American Institute for Cancer Research (aicr.org)

Cancer Resources, The Physicians Committee (www.cancerproject.org)

Articles

For further detailed information, you can access the following study abstracts.

Chapter 1:

Natural health products that inhibit angiogenesis: a potential source for investigational new agents to treat cancer: https://www.ncbi.nlm.nih.gov/pmc/articles/PMC1891166/

Chapter 2:

Interventions for promoting habitual exercise in people living with and beyond cancer:
https://www.ncbi.nlm.nih.gov/pubmed/24065550

Effects and moderators of exercise on quality of life and physical function in patients with cancer: an individual patient data meta-analysis of 34 RCTs:
https://www.ncbi.nlm.nih.gov/pubmed/28006694

Association of "weekend warrior" and other leisure time physical activity patterns with risks for all-cause, cardiovascular disease, and cancer mortality:
https://www.ncbi.nlm.nih.gov/pubmed/28097313

Dose-response effects of aerobic exercise on quality of life in postmenopausal women: results from the breast cancer and exercise trial in Alberta (BETA): https://www.ncbi.nlm.nih.gov/pubmed/27837524

Exercise interventions on health-related quality of life for people with cancer during active treatment: https://www.ncbi.nlm.nih.gov/pubmed/22895974

Alternative exercise traditions in cancer rehabilitation: https://www.ncbi.nlm.nih.gov/pubmed/27912996

Exercise-induced biochemical changes and their potential influence on cancer: a scientific review: https://www.ncbi.nlm.nih.gov/pubmed/27993842

Physical activity during and after adjuvant treatment for breast cancer:

https://www.ncbi.nlm.nih.gov/pubmed/28008778

The effect of exercise on body composition and bone mineral density in breast cancer survivors taking aromatase inhibitors: https://www.ncbi.nlm.nih.gov/pubmed/28026901

Can supervised exercise prevent treatment toxicity in patients with prostate cancer initiating androgen-deprivation therapy: a randomised controlled trial: https://www.ncbi.nlm.nih.gov/pubmed/24467669

Effects of exercise on treatment-related adverse effects for patients with prostate cancer receiving androgen-deprivation therapy: a systematic review: https://www.ncbi.nlm.nih.gov/pubmed/24344218

Inflammation, cardiometabolic markers, and functional changes in men with prostate cancer. A randomized controlled trial of a 12-month exercise program: https://www.ncbi.nlm.nih.gov/pubmed/28075422

Effects of exercise on sleep problems in breast cancer patients receiving radiotherapy: a randomized clinical trial: https://www.ncbi.nlm.nih.gov/pubmed/28181128

Exercise interventions to reduce cancer-related fatigue and improve health-related quality of life in cancer patients: https://www.ncbi.nlm.nih.gov/pubmed/28181972

Exercise interventions on health-related quality of life for cancer survivors: https://www.ncbi.nlm.nih.gov/pubmed/22895961

Impact of acute intermittent exercise on natural killer cells in breast cancer survivors: https://www.ncbi.nlm.nih.gov/pubmed/25873292

Effects of exercise on markers of oxidative stress: an ancillary analysis of the Alberta Physical Activity and Breast Cancer Prevention Trial: https://www.ncbi.nlm.nih.gov/pubmed/27900199

Cancer treatment induced metabolic syndrome: Improving outcome with lifestyle: https://www.ncbi.nlm.nih.gov/pubmed/27931830

Changes in insulin resistance indicators, IGFs, and adipokines in a year-long trial of aerobic exercise in postmenopausal women:
https://www.ncbi.nlm.nih.gov/pubmed/21482635

Effects of exercise intervention in breast cancer patients: is mobile health (mHealth) with pedometer more effective than conventional program using brochure?:
https://www.ncbi.nlm.nih.gov/pubmed/27933450

Efficacy, feasibility, and acceptability of a novel technology-based intervention to support physical activity in cancer survivors:
https://www.ncbi.nlm.nih.gov/pubmed/27957621

Exercise training intensity prescription in breast cancer survivors: validity of current practice and specific recommendations:
https://www.ncbi.nlm.nih.gov/pubmed/25711667

Randomized controlled trial of the effects of high intensity and low-to-moderate intensity exercise on physical fitness and fatigue in cancer survivors: results of the Resistance and Endurance exercise After ChemoTherapy (REACT) study:
https://www.ncbi.nlm.nih.gov/pubmed/26515383

Moderate-intensity exercise reduces fatigue and improves mobility in cancer survivors: a systematic review and meta-regression:
https://www.ncbi.nlm.nih.gov/pubmed/26996098

Effect of walking on circadian rhythms and sleep quality of patients with lung cancer: a randomised controlled trial: https://www.ncbi.nlm.nih.gov/pubmed/27811855

Impact of moderate intensity aerobic exercise on chemotherapy-induced anemia in elderly women with breast cancer: A randomized controlled clinical trial: https://www.ncbi.nlm.nih.gov/pubmed/27872759

A dance intervention for cancer survivors and their partners (RHYTHM):
https://www.ncbi.nlm.nih.gov/pubmed/28070770

Yoga for improving health-related quality of life, mental health and cancer-related symptoms in women diagnosed with breast cancer:
https://www.ncbi.nlm.nih.gov/pubmed/28045199

Yoga management of breast cancer-related lymphoedema: a randomised controlled pilot-trial: https://www.ncbi.nlm.nih.gov/pubmed/24980836

Bone mineral density, balance performance, balance self-efficacy, and falls in breast cancer survivors with and without qigong training:
https://www.ncbi.nlm.nih.gov/pubmed/28050925

Participation in and adherence to physical exercise after completion of primary cancer treatment: https://www.ncbi.nlm.nih.gov/pubmed/27612561

Higher-intensity exercise helps cancer survivors remain

motivated:
https://www.ncbi.nlm.nih.gov/pubmed/26586495

Effect of aerobic exercise on cancer-associated cognitive
impairment: A proof-of-concept RCT:
https://www.ncbi.nlm.nih.gov/pubmed/28075038

Nutrition therapy with high intensity interval training to
improve prostate cancer-related fatigue in men on
androgen deprivation therapy: a study protocol:
https://www.ncbi.nlm.nih.gov/pubmed/28049525

A 3-week multimodal intervention involving high-
intensity interval training in female cancer survivors: a
randomized controlled trial:
https://www.ncbi.nlm.nih.gov/pubmed/26869680

High shear stresses under exercise condition destroy
circulating tumor cells in a microfluidic system:
https://www.ncbi.nlm.nih.gov/pubmed/28054593

Circulatory shear flow alters the viability and
proliferation of circulating colon cancer cells:
https://www.ncbi.nlm.nih.gov/pmc/articles/PMC48917
68/

Significantly greater reduction in breast cancer mortality
from post-diagnosis running than walking:
http://onlinelibrary.wiley.com/doi/10.1002/ijc.28740/ful
l

Triathlon training for women breast cancer survivors:

feasibility and initial efficacy:
https://www.ncbi.nlm.nih.gov/pubmed/28012121

Resistance training interventions across the cancer control continuum: a systematic review of the implementation of resistance training principles:
https://www.ncbi.nlm.nih.gov/pubmed/27986761

Evaluation of resistance training to improve muscular strength and body composition in cancer patients undergoing neoadjuvant and adjuvant therapy: a meta-analysis:
https://www.ncbi.nlm.nih.gov/pubmed/28054255

Progressive strength training to prevent LYmphoedema in the first year after breast CAncer - the LYCA feasibility study:
https://www.ncbi.nlm.nih.gov/pubmed/28084150

Is it safe and efficacious for women with lymphedema secondary to breast cancer to lift heavy weights during exercise: a randomised controlled trial:
https://www.ncbi.nlm.nih.gov/pubmed/23604998

Impact of resistance training in cancer survivors: a meta-analysis:
https://www.ncbi.nlm.nih.gov/pubmed/23669878

Weight training is not harmful for women with breast cancer-related lymphoedema: a systematic review:
https://www.ncbi.nlm.nih.gov/pubmed/25086730

Effects of physical activity on systemic oxidative/DNA status in breast cancer survivors:
https://www.ncbi.nlm.nih.gov/pubmed/28123580

"We're All in the Same Boat": A review of the benefits of dragon boat racing for women living with breast cancer:
https://www.ncbi.nlm.nih.gov/pubmed/22811743

Survivor dragon boating: a vehicle to reclaim and enhance life after treatment for breast cancer:
https://www.ncbi.nlm.nih.gov/pubmed/17364976

The comparative effectiveness of a team-based versus group-based physical activity intervention for cancer survivors:
https://www.ncbi.nlm.nih.gov/pubmed/21932141

Moderate load eccentric exercise; a distinct novel training modality:
https://www.ncbi.nlm.nih.gov/pubmed/27899894

Greater strength gains after training with accentuated eccentric than traditional isoinertial loads in already strength-trained men:
https://www.ncbi.nlm.nih.gov/pubmed/27199764

Nature-based experiences and health of cancer survivors:
https://www.ncbi.nlm.nih.gov/pubmed/25160991

Tailoring exercise interventions to comorbidities and treatment-induced adverse effects in patients with early stage breast cancer undergoing chemotherapy: a

framework to support clinical decisions:
https://www.ncbi.nlm.nih.gov/pubmed/28054496

Clinical approach for patient-centered physical activity assessment and interventions:
https://cjon.ons.org/cjon/20/6/supplement/clinical-approach-patient-centered-physical-activity-assessment-and

A feasibility study related to inactive cancer survivors compared with non-cancer controls during aerobic exercise training:
https://www.ncbi.nlm.nih.gov/pubmed/27928204

A feasibility study related to inactive cancer survivors compared with non-cancer controls during aerobic exercise training:
https://www.ncbi.nlm.nih.gov/pubmed/27928204

Chapter 3:

Is there a role for carbohydrate restriction in the treatment and prevention of cancer?
https://www.ncbi.nlm.nih.gov/pmc/articles/PMC3267662/

Ketogenic diets as an adjuvant cancer therapy: History and potential mechanism
https://www.ncbi.nlm.nih.gov/pmc/articles/PMC4215472/

Warburg Effect or reverse Warburg Effect? A review of cancer metabolism:
https://www.karger.com/Article/FullText/375435

Role of life-style and dietary habits in risk of cancer among seventh-day Adventists, Cancer Res 1975;35:3513 – 22

Health effects of vegan diets:
http://ajcn.nutrition.org/content/89/5/1627S.full

Vegetarian diets and the incidence of cancer in a low-risk population:
http://cebp.aacrjournals.org/content/22/2/286

Prolonged nightly fasting and breast cancer prognosis:
http://jamanetwork.com/journals/jamaoncology/article-abstract/2506710

The impact of religious fasting on human health:
https://www.ncbi.nlm.nih.gov/pmc/articles/PMC2995774/

Chapter 4:

Voluntary activation of the sympathetic nervous system and attenuation of the innate immune response in humans: http://www.pnas.org/content/111/20/7379

Stress management techniques: evidence-based procedures that reduce stress and promote health:
http://www.hsj.gr/medicine/stress-management-techniques-evidencebased-procedures-that-reduce-stress-and-promote-health.php?aid=3429

Facilitation and inhibition of breathing during changes in emotion: https://link.springer.com/chapter/10.1007/978-

4-431-67901-1_14

Chapter 5:

BC Wolverton; WL Douglas; K Bounds (July 1989). A study of interior landscape plants for indoor air pollution abatement: report. NASA. NASA-TM-108061.

Wolverton, B. C., et al. Interior landscape plants for indoor air pollution abatement: final report. NASA. September, 1989. pp 11-12.

Orwell, R.; Wood, R.; Tarran, J.; Torpy, F.; Burchett, M. (2004). "Removal of Benzene by the Indoor Plant/Substrate Microcosm and Implications for Air Quality". Water, Air, & Soil Pollution. 157 (1–4): 193–207.

Endocrine disruptor induction of epigenetic transgenerational inheritance of disease: https://www.ncbi.nlm.nih.gov/pubmed/25088466

Environmentally induced epigenetic transgenerational inheritance of reproductive disease: https://www.ncbi.nlm.nih.gov/pubmed/26510870

Genome-wide locations of potential epimutations associated with environmentally induced epigenetic transgenerational inheritance of disease using a sequential machine learning prediction approach: https://www.ncbi.nlm.nih.gov/pubmed/26571271

Developmental origins of epigenetic transgenerational

inheritance:
https://www.ncbi.nlm.nih.gov/pubmed/27390622

Differential DNA methylation regions in adult human sperm following adolescent chemotherapy: potential for epigenetic inheritance:
https://www.ncbi.nlm.nih.gov/pubmed/28146567

Environmental chemicals in an urban population of pregnant women and their newborns from San Francisco:
https://www.ncbi.nlm.nih.gov/pubmed/27700069

Transport of persistent organic pollutants across the human placenta:
https://www.ncbi.nlm.nih.gov/pubmed/24486968

Prenatal triclosan exposure and cord blood immune system biomarkers:
https://www.ncbi.nlm.nih.gov/pubmed/27167448

Chemical analyses of 10 umbilical cord blood samples were conducted by AXYS Analytical Services (Sydney, BC) and Flett Research Ltd. (Winnipeg, MB).

Environmental Working Group analysis of tests of 10 umbilical cord blood samples conducted by AXYS Analytical Services (Sydney, BC) and Flett Research Ltd. (Winnipeg, MB)

Chapter 6:

The Nocebo Effect: Negative Thoughts Can Harm Your Health:

https://www.psychologytoday.com/blog/owning-pink/201308/the-nocebo-effect-negative-thoughts-can-harm-your-health

Positive thinking: Stop negative self-talk to reduce stress: http://www.mayoclinic.org/healthy-lifestyle/stress-management/in-depth/positive-thinking/art-20043950

The Role of Gratitude in Breast Cancer: Its Relationships with Post-traumatic Growth, Psychological Well-Being and Distress: https://link.springer.com/article/10.1007/s10902-012-9330-x

Gratitude and the Science of Positive Psychology: https://books.google.com/books?hl=en&lr=&id=2Cr5rP8jOnsC&oi=fnd&pg=PA459&dq=gratitude+and+health&ots=elC0fyEDWW&sig=iqMhFCJ6skqOQIKhrNMDwJamUsg#v=onepage&q=gratitude%20and%20health&f=false

Gratitude and Well Being: The Benefits of Appreciation: https://www.ncbi.nlm.nih.gov/pmc/articles/PMC3010965/

The Effect of the Bonny Method of Guided Imagery and Music on the Mood and Life Quality of Cancer Patients: https://academic.oup.com/jmt/article-abstract/38/1/51/893547

Relaxation and imagery in the treatment of breast cancer: http://www.bmj.com/content/297/6657/1169

The effect of hypnotic-guided imagery on psychological well-being and immune function in patients with prior breast cancer:
http://www.sciencedirect.com/science/article/pii/S0022399902004099

Efficacy of relaxation training and guided imagery in reducing the aversiveness of cancer chemotherapy:
http://psycnet.apa.org/record/1982-28546-001

Effects of guided imagery and music (GIM) therapy on mood and cortisol in healthy adults:
http://psycnet.apa.org/record/1997-05310-011

Weaving a circle: A relaxation program using imagery and music:
https://search.proquest.com/openview/26a77197acde88 8a36a6bd430491f53c/1?pq-origsite=gscholar&cbl=31334

Otto, A. K., Szczesny, E. C., Soriano, E. C., Laurenceau, J., & Siegel, S. D. (2016). Effects of a randomized gratitude intervention on death-related fear of recurrence in breast cancer survivors. Health Psychology, 35, 1320-1328. doi:10.1037/hea0000400

The effect of hypnotic-guided imagery on psychological well-being and immune function in patients with prior breast cancer:
https://www.ncbi.nlm.nih.gov/pubmed/12479996

Guided imagery effects on chemotherapy induced nausea and vomiting in Iranian breast cancer patients:

http://www.sciencedirect.com/science/article/pii/S1744
388116300561

Chapter 7:

Integrative Medicine Vol. 15, No. 1 February 2016
https://www.aihm.org/wp-content/uploads/The-
Academy-of-Integrative-Health-and-Medicine-and-the-
Evolution-of-Integrative-Medicine-Practice-Education-
and-Fellowships.pdf   http://drjefftarrant.com/wp-
content/uploads/2015/10/sLORETA-changes-in-
specific-brain-regions-during-meditation-on-Twin-
Hearts-flyer_en.pdf

The unique brain anatomy of meditation practitioners:
alterations in cortical gyrification:
https://www.ncbi.nlm.nih.gov/pmc/articles/PMC32899
49/

What Science Tells Us About Meditation on Twin Hearts
and Our Brain:
http://static1.squarespace.com/static/55a1e4a2e4b0ffb2
0cede22d/t/56d89b6286db4376b82aac75/14570361304
95/What+Science+Tells+Us+About+MTH.pdf

Rapid changes in histone deacetylases and inflammatory
gene   expression   in   expert   meditators:
https://www.ncbi.nlm.nih.gov/pmc/articles/PMC40391
94/

Yogic meditation reverses NF-κB and IRF-related
transcriptome dynamics in leukocytes of family
dementia caregivers in a randomized controlled trial:

https://www.ncbi.nlm.nih.gov/pubmed/22795617

Reduced stress and inflammatory responsiveness in experienced meditators compared to a matched healthy control group:
https://www.ncbi.nlm.nih.gov/pubmed/26970711

Pain sensitivity and analgesic effects of mindful states in Zen meditators: a cross-sectional study:
https://www.ncbi.nlm.nih.gov/pubmed/19073756

The effects of brief mindfulness meditation training on experimentally induced pain:
https://www.ncbi.nlm.nih.gov/pubmed/19853530

Gen Hosp Psychiatry. 1982 Apr;4(1):33-47.

Mindfulness meditation improves emotion regulation and reduces drug abuse:
https://www.ncbi.nlm.nih.gov/pubmed/27306725

Circuitry of self-control and its role in reducing addiction:
https://www.ncbi.nlm.nih.gov/pubmed/26235449

Brief meditation training induces smoking reduction:
https://www.ncbi.nlm.nih.gov/pubmed/23918376

JAMA Psychiatr. 2014;71:547–556. doi: 10.1001/jamapsychiatry.2013.4546. [PMC free article] [PubMed] [Cross Ref]

Meditation or exercise for preventing acute respiratory infection: a randomized controlled trial:

https://www.ncbi.nlm.nih.gov/pmc/articles/PMC33922
93/

http://www.medscape.com/viewarticle/788539

Relaxation response induces temporal transcriptome
changes in energy metabolism, insulin secretion and
inflammatory pathways:
https://www.ncbi.nlm.nih.gov/pmc/articles/PMC36411
12/

Fifteen minutes of chair-based yoga postures or guided
meditation performed in the office can elicit a relaxation
response:
https://www.ncbi.nlm.nih.gov/pmc/articles/PMC32650
94/

The effectiveness and cost-effectiveness of mindfulness-
based cognitive therapy compared with maintenance
antidepressant treatment in the prevention of depressive
relapse/recurrence: results of a randomised controlled
trial (the PREVENT study):
https://www.ncbi.nlm.nih.gov/pubmed/26379122

Meditation programs for psychological stress and well-
being: a systematic review and meta-analysis:
https://www.ncbi.nlm.nih.gov/pubmed/24395196/

MAP training: combining meditation and aerobic
exercise reduces depression and rumination while
enhancing synchronized brain activity:
https://www.ncbi.nlm.nih.gov/pubmed/26836414

Neural correlates of mindfulness meditation-related

anxiety relief:
https://www.ncbi.nlm.nih.gov/pmc/articles/PMC40400
88/

Mindfulness meditation and improvement in sleep quality and daytime impairment among older adults with sleep disturbances: a randomized clinical trial: https://www.ncbi.nlm.nih.gov/pubmed/25686304

Sante Ment Que. 2013 Autumn;38(2):19-34. [Review of the effects of mindfulness meditation on mental and physical health and its mechanisms of action]. Ngô TL1.

Mens Sana Monogr. 2008 Jan-Dec; 6(1): 63–80. Neurobiology of Spirituality. E. Mohandas, M.D.

Nature Reviews: Neuroscience. 2015, April(16): 213 - 225. Tang, YY. Britta, K. Posner, M.

The effects of running and meditation on beta-endorphin, corticotropin-releasing hormone and cortisol in plasma, and on mood:
http://www.sciencedirect.com/science/article/pii/03010
5119505118T

Lowering cortisol and CVD risk in postmenopausal women: a pilot study using the transcendental meditation program:
http://onlinelibrary.wiley.com/doi/10.1196/annals.1314.
023/full

Effect of compassion meditation on neuroendocrine, innate immune and behavioral responses to psychosocial

stress:
http://www.sciencedirect.com/science/article/pii/S0306
453008002199

Brown, RP, et al. Sudarshan Kriya yogic breathing in the treatment of stress, anxiety, and depression: part 1- neurophysiologic model. J Altern Complement Med 2005 Apr;11(2):383-4.

Harvard Medical School. Harvard Health Publications. Stress Management: Approaches for preventing and reducing stress. May 2009.

Brown, RP, et al. Yoga breathing, meditation, and longevity. Ann N Y Acad Sci 2009 Aug 1172:54-62.

Katiyar, SK, et al. Role of Pranayama in Rehabilitation of COPD patients—a Randomized Controlled Study. Indian J Allergy Asthma Immunol 2006;20(2):98-104.

Seppala, EM, et al. Breathing-based meditation decreases posttraumatic stress disorder symptoms in US military veterans: a randomized controlled longitudinal study. J Trauma Stress. 2014 Aug;27(4):397-405.

Manoj K. Bhasin, Jeffery A. Dusek, Bei-Hung Chang, Marie G. Joseph, John W. Denninger, Gregory L. Fricchione, Herbert Benson, Towia A. Libermann. Relaxation Response Induces Temporal Transcriptome Changes in Energy Metabolism, Insulin Secretion and Inflammatory Pathways. PLoS ONE, 2013; 8 (5): e62817 DOI: 10.1371/journal.pone.0062817

Integrative Medicine, Vol. 15, No. 1 February 2016: https://www.aihm.org/wp-content/uploads/The-Academy-of-Integrative-Health-and-Medicine-and-the-Evolution-of-Integrative-Medicine-Practice-Education-and-Fellowships.pdf

sLORETA changes in specific brain regions during Meditation on Twin Hearts: Differences between novice and experienced meditators: http://drjefftarrant.com/wp-content/uploads/2015/10/sLORETA-changes-in-specific-brain-regions-during-meditation-on-Twin-Hearts-flyer_en.pdf

Prayer and healing: A medical and scientific perspective on randomized controlled trials: https://www.ncbi.nlm.nih.gov/pmc/articles/PMC2802370/

Meditation, prayer and spiritual healing: the evidence: https://www.ncbi.nlm.nih.gov/pmc/articles/PMC3396089/

Is the spiritual life of cancer patients a resource to be taken into account by professional caregivers from the time of diagnosis?: https://www.ncbi.nlm.nih.gov/pubmed/22495717

What is the evidence for the use of mindfulness-based interventions in cancer care? A review. C Shennan and others. Psychooncology, 2011. Volume 20, Issue 7

Mindfulness-based stress reduction and cancer: a meta-analysis, D Ledesma and H Kumano. Psychooncology,

2009. Volume 18, Issue 6

Randomised controlled trial of mindfulness-based stress reduction (MBSR) for survivors of breast cancer. CA Lengacher and others. Psychooncology, 2009. Volume 16, Issue 6

Mindfulness meditation for oncology patients: a discussion and critical review, MJ Ott and others. Integrative Cancer Therapies, 2006. Volume 5, Issue 2

BACK MATTER

❋——❋——❋

Cancer Proof is a roadmap for anyone wanting to know strategies for overcoming, preventing, and recovering from cancer. *Cancer Proof* tells us:

- why knowing your own body is the key to cancer care

- how much and what type of exercise is best

- the secret to gentle detoxification

- strategies to cleanse for cancer prevention and to recover from cancer treatments

- how to stop doing unspecific diet programs and discover your ideal diet

- the healing power of your mind

- going deeper than cell biology by diving into the soul of illness and healing

After Dr. Heather Paulson's personal experience of losing her father to colon cancer, followed by her husband being diagnosed with lymphoma she knew that it was time to quit the path of study she had started down, and dive into the causes and prevention of cancer.

Her journey from marine biologist to cancer physician has revealed many tools that anyone can apply to their lives to help them become *Cancer Proof.* She gathered these tools together in this book to help you on your journey to living a *Cancer Proof* life.

26068246R00161

Made in the USA
San Bernardino, CA
15 February 2019